HOMEO REMEDIES

Homeopathic Cures for Common Diseases

Dr. David Dancu, N.D.

FULL CIRCLE

HOMEOPATHIC REMEDIES
© All Rights Reserved, 1998
First Paperback Edition, 1998
ISBN 81-7621-022-6

Published by arrangement with Gaia Midia A.G.

 Published by FULL CIRCLE
18-19, Dilshad Garden
G.T. Road, Delhi-110095
Tel: 2297792, 93, 94 Fax: 2282332

Designing, Typesetting
   Print Production: **SCANSET**

18-19 Dilshad Garden, G.T. Road, Delhi-110 095
Tel: 228 2467, 229 7792, 93, 94   Fax: 228 2332

Printed at Nutech Photolithographers, Delhi-110095

PRINTED IN INDIA

Acknowledgements

To my life partner and wife Anne, for the many hours of guidance, love, support and freedom to write and play golf. Her editing and aesthetic balance helped decipher my notes, thoughts and concerns.

To my son Joshua who unknowingly relinquished some of our morning time together so that I could write.

To Robin Murphy, who freely shared his knowledge and homeopathic gifts.

To Julie Clemens, who initially saw the value in my work.

To my students and patients who aked me to share my teaching and experience with others.

To Maruti Seidman for encouraging me to golf and relax.

To Denny Johnson, whose words of wisdom and caring allowed me to discover a deeper purpose.

To Mark Hochwender for his guidance, suggestions and friendship.

To Jack Hofer, my publisher, for his uncanny ability to find just the right word while bringing my manuscript to life.

And finally, to all those individuals interested in learning, growing and healing through the wonders of homeopathy.

This book discusses the theories and principles of homeopathy and has been written as an educational guide for health care practitioners and laypersons. It is not intended to replace the services of a health care provider or to act as a diagnostic tool. Any therapy undertaken for physical or emotional ailments should be properly supervised by an experienced provider. The author and publisher disclaim any responsibility arising from the use of information contained within this book. Responsibility for using the material contained herein is solely that of the reader.

If you feel you or others have a medical or psychological problem, consult with a competent health care provider before pursuing any of the information in this book.

Contents

Introduction

I first heard about homeopathy in 1986. And even on hearing it, I was not sure what it meant. Within the next several years the field and its deeper meaning became clearer to me as I pursued alternative healing ideas through education and clinical practice.

My desire was to uncover a natural, safe and effective healing process to help family and friends. I did not want to work with many of the techniques and suppressive ideas embraced by western medicine.

I read everything I could find on the subject of natural healing and homeopathy. My search filled me with questions and doubts. Questions remain, as my study of homeopathy continues. Understanding has grown with each patient I have seen and with each student I teach.

There were no homeopathic schools when I began my studies. I was self-taught with the aid of homeopathic groups interested in pursuing a course of education. The Pacific Academy of Homeopathic Medicine in Berkeley, California was my first experience with organized study. The Academy is a wonderful organization that sponsors international homeopathic teachers and weekend lectures.

I had the good fortune to study with Dr. Francesco Eizayaga, George Vithoulkas, Robin Murphy, Sheiligh Creasy, Dr. Vasillas Ghegas, Andre Saine, Dr. Paul Herscu, Vega Rozenberg, David Warkenton and many others. Each was a blessing in his or her own right, and my experience grew and tools for understanding homeopathy blossomed.

These homeopaths use differrent techniques to analyze and interpret their cases. Throughout this book, I have tried to include as many pieces of information as I could from each of my teachers. Anyone interested in pursuing a career in homeopathy must discover what aspects to use in their practice and what feels most comfortable in his or her approach. The material in *Homeopathic Vibrations* is a guide to help you in understanding the field of homeopathy.

Over the years, I have taught hundreds of students and seen thousands of patients. Each experience has provided a level of joy and reward I could not have predicted. When several students suggested that I write about my teaching and education, I thought about it for years and ultimately decided to write *Homeopathic Vibrations*.

Many books have been written by accomplished homeopaths about materia medica, pathology, educational courses, clinical applications, philosophy and everyday use of remedies. However, none of them seemed to create a guide for a good understanding of basic homeopathic concepts.

I do not pretend that this work is by any means complete, yet I find that it does accomplish one of many goals: To have an easy reference work about Dr. Hahnemann's (the founder of homeopathy) philosophies and ideals.

I have chosen to include some specific illnesses and related remedies, both for acute and chronic problems, as a guide or starting point. I originally intended to write this book specifically for homeopathic students or those interested in learning about homeopathy. Part way through, I changed my intent to include issues for anyone wanting to use homeopathic remedies.

I welcome your ideas, suggestions or constructive comments. My address is listed at the end of the book.

A few notes about the format. Each succeeding chapter builds on the previous one. This establishes a good foundation for understanding homeopathy and its complex approach to healing. Obviously, there is repetition in order to accomplish a deeper grasp of the material. Each of us learns differently and I hope that the repeated information addresses different learning techniques.

Several chapters can be used for specific illnesses and Chapter Six on Materia Medica can give you some insight into remedy keynotes.

Introduction

The material I am presenting is taken from many sources, including lectures, books, research, personal experiences and ideas, questions from students and patients, homeopathic software programs and my own meditations.

It is not intended that this material replace professional diagnosis nor eliminate the need to see a health care provider. The information contained in this book is for education, not the practice of medicine.

This is a source for homeopaths as well as those interested in working with their families or friends in using homeopathic principles and remedies.

If you wish to learn about and use homeopathy, you need two books: a repertory and a materia medica. Remedies can be powerful, yet when used properly, and with accepted principles, can be quite safe and effective.

David A. Dancu, N.D.
Boulder, Colorado

Chapter One

History: The Early Stages

Homeopathy is unique in the annuls of medicine, for it demands intention, attention, interrogation, discovery and compassion. It is far removed from standard medical practices, and rightly so. The basics of homeopathy appear simple, but they take a long time to master.

There are rock climbers and scuba divers who can climb or swim, but without the proper training and equipment, their experiences remain limited and unrewarding. Homeopathic experiences also remain unrewarding and limited without a foundation in the principles of procedure and philosophy.

The term homeopathy is derived from the Greek words, *homeos* and *pathos*, which mean *similar suffering*. Hippocrates' Law of Similars best summarizes the basic concept of homeopathy:

"When a natural substance is given to a healthy individual, symptoms will arise; when that same substance is ingested by someone who is ill with similar symptoms, it acts as a curative."

Webster's 10th Collegiate Dictionary defines homeopathy as: "a system of medical practice that treats a disease especially by the administration of minute doses of a remedy that would in healthy persons produce symptoms similar to those of the disease."

In 1810, Dr. Samuel Hahnemann, M.D., composed the word homeopathy, after he had intentionally taken an herb to find out how it affected him.

The herb was Chinchona Bark and he decided to take it after reading about its remarkable results with malaria cases. Hahnemann wanted to learn why specific malaria symptoms were eliminated after taking this bitter herb. Despite not having any symptoms of malaria or being ill in any way, he chose to ingest the herb to discover what symptoms might arise.

Much to his amazement, he developed the typical symptoms of malaria. The symptoms dissipated after several hours and his health returned. He repeated the procedure several times. And it was from a series of experiments with different substances that Dr. Hahnemann determined the accuracy and validity of Hippocrates' theories. Hence, homéopathy as a medicine and a science had its beginning.

To further document these theories, he enlisted fellow German doctors, friends and family members to assist with additional *provings*. This is the term he used to describe symptoms that arise in an individual after taking a natural substance. All symptoms were contrasted between preexisting ones and new ones. Then each specific symptom was transcribed to maintain an exact record. For example, after taking Chinchona these symptoms arose and were recorded:

"Sensitivity to touch; aversion to being looked at; inability to think; fixed ideas; anxiety felt at 8:00 p.m.; congestive headache with throbbing sensation, like hammers; loss of appetite; flatulance; painless diarrhea; periodicity of ailments; shaking chills; fever; vomiting and sweat with thirst."

This is just a brief list of a larger symptom picture derived from ingesting Chinchona Bark, but it gives some understanding of what can occur in a proving.

As Hahnemann's ideas slowly spread throughout Germany, his provings set the stage for further healing and a reduction in side effects or poisonings. Others took up the call to reform "medicine" and eliminate the problems caused by medical procedures in the 1700's.

The process was not a simple one, but rather one of time-consuming effort and commitment. Provings alone were not enough, as the herbs, plants, minerals, flowers and even poisons needed to be diluted to avoid ill effects and create a safe yet powerful means of healing. These substances are called *homeopathic remedies* and when given to a person with various symptoms, aid them in the recovery of his or her health.

Dr. Hahnemann's work was not rapidly accepted, despite its effective results with both epidemics and disease. Another German, Dr. Constantine Hering, set out to disprove homeopathy. To his surprise, however, he discovered that Hahnemann's principles created a natural means of healing without side effects. There were effects in the form of a release of older symptoms, but no side effects such as is found with current medications and drugs. Hering's research totally altered his perspective on medicine. He went on to become one of Hahnemann's most famous followers, a man who authored numerous books, established schools in the United States and practiced homeopathy in Philiadelphia after leaving Germany.

So why did Hahnemann begin this difficult research into natural healing? Being an authority on toxicology and metal poisoning, along with his medical degree and versatility with many languages, Dr. Hahnemann was considered an expert in several fields. Nonetheless, he was disillusioned with the medical practices being used at that time. They included bloodletting, mercury poisoning, cupping and leaching.

Hahnemann could no longer accept these forms of "medicine" as he felt they were barbaric and of little long-term value. When he quit his medical practice in protest, he began translating foreign medical books to support his growing family. It was while translating Cullen's Materia Medica, that he began to question Cullen's proposition that Cinchona Bark cured malaria because it was a bitter herb. Hahnemann knew that no other bitter herb would cure malaria in quite the same manner and so began his experiments.

He started collating his research about poisons, plants, herbs and medicines. The process included ancient writings and observations from toxicology and herbology. These old documents proved unclear and quite inadequate. So, he painstakingly kept records of his provings and data to maintain an exact account of the results. Because of jealous and narrow-minded men of his time, Hahnemann was banned from the practice of medicine. He left Germany to further establish homeopathy and its principles wherever they would be accepted.

Hahnemann published the first edition of his Organon in 1810, a compilation of his ideas and philosophies to help guide others in the formulation of homeopathic principles. He stated:

"The highest ideal of therapy is to restore health rapidly, gently, permanently; to remove and destroy the whole disease in the shortest, surest, least harmful way, according to clearly comprehensible principles."

As he continued with his experiments and worked with the remedies, Hahnemann refined and evolved his procedures while creating new preparations and administering remedies to the ill. He wrote five additional editions during his lifetime, but the sixth was not published until many years after his death. The original manuscript from the sixth edition had been in the possession of his second wife Melanie, and was not available for publication.

Melanie had attempted to sell the work on several occasions but was unable to reach agreement as to price. The sixth edition went undiscovered for decades and was found in an attic in 1920 and published in 1921. It contained new revelations about Hahnemann's last ideas and methods for the use of various remedies. The primary change dealt with LM potencies which reduced aggravations while accelerating the healing process. LM potencies and aggravations are covered in Chapter Two.

The sixth edition was not readily accepted or acknowledged by the homeopathic communities in either Europe or the United States. The changes made by Hahnemann from the fifth edition were consequential and dramatic. Even today, although accepted as his actual changes and additions, many homeopaths do not use his last known theories. They feel that the results achieved without the later changes are just as effective and permanent. Therefore, these particular homeopaths are reluctant to consider the value of Hahnemann's final writings.

Besides writing six Organons, Hahnemann had over 1500 pages of cases and notes from patients, making up four volumes of information and cures. These four volumes did not include the 470 remedies he published in his own materia medica, which is a compilation of information on symptoms that arose from the provings. The symptoms he described covered mental, emotional, physical and pathological findings, along with the essence of the remedy. His materia medica also included clinical experiences from cured cases, which helped verify many specific patient provings.

When he was 80 years old, Hahnemann moved to Paris with his second wife, Melanie. His work prospered and he was granted special rights to practice medicine and homeopathy there.

It wasn't until 1825 that homeopathy was introduced to the United States by Dr. Gram. He was a former student of Dr. Lund, who had been directly taught by Hahnemann. The practice of homeopathy did not require medical licensure at the time and was primarily used by herbologists. German communities in the United States were strong advocates of Hahnemann's theories. In 1833, Dr. Hering came from Europe to establish the first homeopathic medical school in Philadelphia. The success of this new and effective means of treatment spread quickly.

By the 1880's in America, there were 20 homeopathic medical colleges, 100 hospitals and one of every five medical doctors was a homeopath. As medicine changed, scientific research began to establish different forms of treatment, diagnosis and analysis. The American Medical Association was founded in part to stem the growth of homeopathy. It went so far as to ban doctors connected in any way to homeopathic practices and prohibited its members from even consulting with homeopaths. Most of the pharmaceutical companies united to eliminate remedies entirely, as their profits were based upon substance weight and homeopathic remedies were minimal in weight.

James Kent, M.D., one of America's most famous homeopaths moved to Philadelphia in the early 1890's. In a little over eight years, he treated more than 30,000 patients. From these cases and his teachings, along with cases and materia medica from other homeopaths, Kent developed his repertory. His Repertory is a compilation of hundreds of thousands of symptoms. He classified the symptoms by headings that included remedies for balancing those symptoms. The repertory was an enormous undertaking, consuming years of his life.

Since it was first published in 1897, *Kents' Repertory* has been used by homeopaths all over the world for locating specific symptoms.

In his preface to the repertory, Kent states:

"It has been built from all sources and is a compilation of all useful symptoms recorded in the fundamental works of our Materia Medica, as well as from notes of our ablest practitioners. Unverified symptoms have been omitted... when there was doubt as to consistency. Clinical matters have been given a place... where consistent with the nature of the remedy."

In 1910, the Flexner Report was commissioned by the government to evaluate conditions of various medical schools in the United States. The purpose was to determine the type of education being provided in order to improve medical training while establishing standardized procedures. Nonorthodox procedures were condemned or disregarded and the Flexner report was critical of most existing schools, including many homeopathic ones. The report recommended that schools without established standards be closed or denied further funding.

History: The Early Stages

Homeopathic medical schools did not fit the standard medical educational approach to pathology or biochemistry. As a result, homeopathic medical schools were unable to obtain funding to continue. Homeopathy declined considerably and without Kent's followers, it would have died completely in the United States. Homeopathy was not seen as modern or scientific, falling out-of-favor with society because of its unconventional approach.

To find some relationship with the medicine of the day, many homeopaths began treating disease with homeopathic remedies, disregarding the person and focusing on the illness. The results were minimal at best, and patients began to distrust the efficacy of the treatment. Contributing to the decline of homeopathy was the apparent success of scientific medical procedures.

For over 50 years, the practice of homeopathy in the United States was limited to lay practitioners and alternative oriented groups. Remedies were difficult to obtain and books or education were almost impossible to find.

In the early 1970's, a group of doctors, seeking alternatives to the suppressive and often ineffective therapies of orthodox medicine, rediscovered the teachings of Hahnemann. European homeopaths had continued with Hahnemann's theories and provings, allowing the art and science of homeopathy to grow and prosper there.

Homeopaths such as George Vithoulkas from Greece and Dr. Francisco Eizayaga from South America were brought to the United States to instruct and educate anyone interested in learning about Hahnemann's work. Several doctors spent years in Greece studying and practicing with Vithoulkas. Through their inspiration, homeopathy began a revitalization in the United States, which continues today.

Established European homeopathic pharmaceutical companies, have had enormous success in the United States, increasing their sales incrementally over the past decade. They have established U.S. companies to support the growing need and have been joined by many local companies to provide remedies on request.

Many people have turned to homeopathy with lasting results. Information about this success is being distributed through magazines, books, radio and television productions and educational seminars.

There is a rich, vibrant history related to homeopathy, one filled with safe, natural healing techniques. Over one-third of the world's population uses some form of homeopathic medicine or alternative healing means. And, the number increases daily because of the permanent and effective results.

The philosophies, techniques, ideas and tools necessary to use and establish a sound homeopathic foundation are presented in the following chapters. This knowledge will strongly impact your life and allow you to take a greater responsibility for your own healing and health.

Chapter Two

Principles and Philosophy: The Foundation

Both the fifth and sixth editions of Hahnemann's Organon reflect his insight into the principles and philosophy of homeopathy. Each of these works creates a deeper understanding of Dr. Hahnemann's thoughts, ideas, perspectives and commitment to enhancing the ideals of his life's work.

The essence of his Organon writings can be described as follows:

"The like remedy, the single drug, the smallest dose, the infrequent dose, noninterference with the organism's vital reactions, occasional initial and minor aggravation and potentization of the remedy.

To cure mildly, rapidly and permanently, choose in every case of disease, a remedy which can itself produce a similar affection."

The intricacy of these paragraphs requires additional elaboration, as they make up the basis for all homeopathic study. By reviewing the unique components in greater depth, a clearer picture of Hahnemann's theories can be developed.

First, is *the like remedy* which describes specific remedy selections based solely upon that individual's totality. As defined by Hahnemann, the word *totality* encompasses symptoms, pathology, personality, trauma and inherited tendencies. The *like remedy* is also referred to as the remedy most similar to the person's present symptoms.

An example might be helpful in understanding a person's symptoms and their presenting picture. The following symptoms were described by a woman who came to see me with intense headaches. She had:

1. Migraine headaches, coming on just before her period.

2. Arthritis in her joints, especially relating to the left side upper extremities.
3. Chronic runny nose that was worse in the morning.
4. Irritability, especially over minor things.
5. Compulsive tendencies.
6. Fear of commitment in her relationships.
7. Insomnia caused her to awaken consistently at 3 a.m.
8. She was highly motivated, driven and ambitious.
9. She was very sensitive to noises, odors and cigarette smoke.

This only describes a portion of the symptom picture, but it provides some idea of her disharmony. The symptoms can be located in *Kent's Repertory*, with various remedies described under each symptom. The best remedy is based on all of these symptoms. Many remedies reflect the above symptom picture, but what the totality truly represents is the whole person, not just illness or pathology. Symptoms are the body's best attempt at healing and its the overall pattern of the symptoms that provide a clear direction to the *like remedy*.

The essence of the person, not only their emotions, will provide the greatest understanding for the choice of a remedy. In the above example, the sensitivity, compulsiveness and fears reflect her psychological essence. Even though migraines may be her main reason for seeking treatment, by working with other aspects of her life, the remedy given can stimulate balance on deeper levels. This results in deeper harmony while eliminating the migraines.

One of the more difficult aspects arises when the person's health does not return quickly. Normally, most chronic disharmonies have been endured for a long time, so it is important to explain the process of healing. With this approach, a person can understand that a lasting cure comes with time. The *like remedy* will fit the whole person and not just their pathology.

Principles and Philosophy: The Foundation

Discovering the similar remedy is like digging a water well. First, a search is made of the land (the interview), then the well is drilled (questions), and water is found (a remedy). But the water may not be palatable (the wrong remedy) so another well is started (another remedy). It may take time to dig deeply enough to reach the core (the essence of the person in relation to the remedy). When it is found, it lasts for a long time and brings satisfaction to the owner (the individual), and the well digger (the homeopath).

The second principle described in the Organon is *the single drug*, which is a bit easier to understand, as it means just what it implies. One remedy is given at a time and in this way, the effects of the remedy can be clearly seen, without having to guess about which remedy is working or which caused an aggravation.

In evaluating the need to repeat or change a remedy, the *single drug* gives the best indication of which direction to take. The key word to remember is wait. Allow the remedy to find its own level of resonance, regardless of time.

With an acute illness, those which are self-limiting, it is not necessary to wait as long for recovery. Often, improvement occurs within four to eight hours after the first dose, sometimes even sooner. If no effect or change of any kind, consider using another remedy.

There are combination remedies on the market today, some of which can be effective for acute illness, but generally, the single, well-chosen remedy will better serve rapid improvement. Some of the combinations have never been proven, either alone or in combination, so the ill effects can be greater than the possible benefits. Combination remedies are not recommended for long-term chronic disharmony. By some coincidence should the combination be effective, there is no way of knowing which single remedy worked or established balance. A possible proving of an unrelated remedy might take place. This could create a deeper disharmony than originally existed. Increased dosing of all the remedies in the combination might be harmful. The harm comes in the form of new symptoms which may arise from a remedy that does not correspond to existing symptoms. The correct single remedy, based on two or three clear symptoms, creates no ill effects. Should there be new or unrelated symptoms after taking a remedy, discontinue it immediately. Because of the general safe nature of remedies, those ill effects will diminish quickly, depending on the potency of the remedy taken.

Hahnemanns' third principle is *the small dose* which reflects the smallest effective dilution needed for each individual. This is called the remedy potency. In Hahnemann's fifth edition of the Organon, potency varied in range from the centesimal to the decimal. Centesimal meaning one to ninety-nine dilution, i.e., one drop of the substance and 99 drops of either distilled water or alcohol. Original substance [mother tincture] and 99 drops is equal to a 1c potency. Potency ranges from 1c to CM, or 100,000c.

Decimal potencies are made by mixing one drop of mother tincture to 9 drops of alcohol or distilled water. This is the X potency and ranges from 1x to 200x, and sometimes higher. C potencies are more often preferred and used by homeopaths. Also, that is what Hahnemann used.

In the sixth edition of the Organon, Hahnemann presented his final ideas about potency preparation, describing the LM potencies. An LM is made from a 3c potency, to which is added 500 drops of water or alcohol, making an LM tincture. From this tincture, one drop is placed on 300 small poppyseed size sugar pellets, making an LM 1. The LM 2 is made from a single poppyseed size pellet of the LM 1 after diluting it in a small amount of water, shaking vigorously, adding grain alcohol and placing one drop on an additional 300 poppyseed pellets. Each succeeding LM potency is prepared in the same way. LM potencies continue from LM 1 to LM 32.

Hahnemann found that when he used LM potencies, the healing process was accelerated, there were fewer aggravations and they acted in a more gentle manner. Not many

homeopaths use LM's, simply because of custom and prefer-
ence, although they are becoming more accepted and understood. With the LM's, there is less need to question which
potency to utilize as the LM 1 is used first, followed by LM 2
and LM 3, as needed.

So, how do we determine the small dose? Each patient is
unique, so individual determination as to dosage is required.
As a general rule, the vitality of an individual is the key factor
for choice. The stronger the vitality then the higher the
potency, up to about a 200c, especially for those just learning
the process of potency and homeopathy. The lower the
vitality, the lower the potency, about a 6c or so. The remedy
is given one time while waiting for a response from the body.
Repetition of the remedy occurs when the remedy begins to
wear off and old symptoms return. There is no need to repeat
the remedy if improvement has held.

Individual vitality is important because of possible potency
overstimulation of the vital force. If a person's energy is low,
then overstimulation may cause an intense aggravation of
symptoms. If, on the other hand, the vital force is strong
despite the illness, lower potencies will only have a short-
term effect. The strength of the vital force is based on energy
and vitality. For instance, should someone have a cold, yet
be full of energy despite a runny nose and sneezing, then
one could assume that their vitality is strong. Regardless of
the energetic make-up of an individual, the right remedy will
have some effect.

Other factors for potency selection include a person's
sensitivity, the type of illness and their willingness to eliminate specific causes or obstacles. These will be addressed in
later chapters.

By using the smallest beneficial dose, aggravations are
minimized and the vital force is sufficiently stimulated to
assist recovery.

Hahnemanns' fourth postulate, *the infrequent dose* signifies
that the remedy is repeated only as necessary. There are no

specific guidelines except for common sense and observation. If someone returns for a follow-up visit after several months and continues to improve, the remedy would not be repeated. Should the improvement only have lasted a few weeks, then consider repeating the remedy at the same potency. Also, reevaluate the case to find out if another remedy may be better suited for long-term results.

Allow the remedy time to help the body in making its adjustments and changes. Some individuals react within days because of their sensitivity, while others may have no reaction for several months. Much depends on the person, the length of the disharmony, certain predispositions, long-term physical or mental trauma or their willingness and desire to remove obstacles that prevent cure.

We are born with the ability to heal and recover health. The vital force helps this process in various ways, including fevers that burn off infection, endorphines that aid in pain relief and an effective immune system to destroy germs and bacteria. These natural healing abilities are altered and diminished by antibiotics, vaccinations, diet, environmental pollution, stress, anger and many other factors. Homeopathy can help restore the body's natural abilities to recover health without side effects or ingestion of suppressive medications.

Orthodox medical practices have varying effects. Certain procedures, such as overuse of antibiotics and unnecessary or premature surgery, requires additional review and evaluation. These types of procedures would better serve society if utilized after homeopathy rather than before.

The fifth doctrine, *non interference with the organism's vital reactions* embodies Hahnemann's ideas on the vital force.

There are several aspects to the vital force, but of primary interest to the homeopath is the body's defense mechanism. This is what assists the vital force in defending against germs, viruses, microorganisms and disease.

Principles and Philosophy: The Foundation

Our body is made up of energy which flows in various patterns, unique to each individual. We take in energy in the form of food and water which allows us to store energy in our bodies. The vital force is the essence of all energy within the body and can be thought of as its master regulator.

A homeopathic remedy is another form of energy. When we can match the energetic similarity of the individual with a homeopathic remedy, we are able to create a resonance between these two components and stimulate balance within the body. This initiates the healing response required for recovery of health.

Hahnemann's philosophy was to eliminate any possible interference with vital responses, such as circulation, respiration or brain function. Accepted healing practices in the 1700's seemed to cause more harm than good, and Hahnemann's desire was to maintain a safe and gentle, yet effective means of restoring health. This was the underlying basis for his life and work.

He accomplished this goal by consistently validating his beliefs through experimentation. Interference with the body's natural ability to heal was reduced by using the minimum dose, the dilution of substances, the potentization of remedies and patience with the body's healing response.

His sixth component, an *occasional initial aggravation* refers to a healing crisis. Actually, it's a release of symptoms that have been previously suppressed, meaning that symptoms which existed in the past may return. Usually, returning symptoms come and go quickly, depending on their previous severity, but there will be some form of aggravation relating to prior symptoms.

Another example may help to clarify what occurs after taking a remedy and an aggravation arises. These initial symptoms were described by a 54-year-old woman who just lost her job after 20 years:

1. Insomnia, anger and resentment.
2. Depression about losing her job.

3. Body aches and muscle soreness.
4. Poor memory, especially short term.
5. Diminished appetite.
6. Low self-esteem
7. Grief with feelings of loneliness.

In analyzing the symptoms presented, the cause of the current disharmony appears to be loss of employment. Poor confidence and loneliness are deeper emotional elements and more constitutional in nature. The term *constitutional* describes the person as a whole combining both acute and chronic illness, as well as the essence of the person. This includes lifelong tendencies, personality and predispositions.

Remedies are selected on the totality of symptoms as much as possible. In this instance, three days after taking the remedy, she calls to say that a skin rash she had as a teenager has returned. This is an aggravation and should last for only a few hours, but it is a good sign that the remedy is working and releasing old suppressed symptoms. If it lasts longer than a few hours or a day, the remedy was given in too high of a potency. This indicates her system was overstimulated.

Several choices can be made to eliminate the aggravation, including antidoting the remedy, reducing the potency of the same remedy and repeating or waiting it out. Generally, waiting is best, unless the symptoms become too intense or remain for a longer time. Antidoting may cause a relapse of both old and current symptoms and can slow or reverse the action of the remedy.

Dr. Hahnemann's attitude toward aggravations reflects his commitment to the time and effort required in choosing both the remedy and the potency. By using the lowest possible potency for effectiveness, aggravations will be minor, of short duration and occasional rather than frequent or severe.

The seventh concept embraced by Hahnemann concerns *potentization of the remedy*. Specifically, this relates to the process of dilution and succussion in a particular manner.

Principles and Philosophy: The Foundation

Remedies are derived from plants, minerals, flowers, herbs, insects, animals, reptiles and actual diseased mucosa. Each remedy is carefully chosen to ensure that it is of the highest quality. This allows pharmaceutical companies to maintain strict standards of reliability for future production.

To eliminate any possibility of toxicity, each remedy is diluted with either distilled water or alcohol. The lower the dilution, from 1c to 12c, the greater the amount of substance in the final product. Beyond a 12c, no physical substance remains, just the energy of the substance.

Energy remains because each dilution is succused, or shaken vigorously 100 times before proceeding to the next dilution. For instance, one drop from the mother tincture of a substance, added to 99 drops of water is succused 100 times by striking the bottle against an object soft enough not to break the glass. This is a 1c potency, from which one drop is taken and added to 99 drops of water and succussed. This is a 2c. Dilutions continue up to 100,000c or CM, with each separate potency being succussed and properly diluted.

Succussions may vary between remedies and production companies, but it is the movement of the liquid solution that establishes the breakdown of the molecules of each substance, not the type of succussion. The energy from the original substance remains in the diluted form of the remedy. This contains the essence of that substance, without any of its toxicity. Most of the pharmaceutical companies making remedies structure the dilutions as follows: 6c; 12c; 30c; 200c; 1m (1000c); 10m; 50m; CM. In between potencies can be obtained, if available, but those described above are the most common ones.

Hahnemann initially used crude substances, along with existing materia medica, to formalize his provings. From these provings, he established his own materia medica. It was also through these provings that he discovered how crude substances were just as harmful as some of the medical practices being used. When he began to experiment with his dilution and succussion ideas, he established potencies through reduction of the amount of substance. This was his means of eliminating disharmony without harm. Dr. Hahnemann found that his dilutions provided beneficial results to patients and provers alike.

Hahnemann compiled and documented his work over several decades, and the question most frequently asked was how the remedies actually work. The question is still asked of homeopaths, none of whom have a definitive answer. Theories abound, but health returns, balance and homeostasis are obtained, yet the complete answer remains elusive. They just work, say some, and why question what has been effective.

In the simplest terms, remedies work because they resonate with the energetic pattern of the individual and stimulate a response from the vital force.

All living things are energy, composed of molecules and atoms. Energy consumes energy to survive, whether its food, water, sunlight or minerals. When energy is in balance, the system works in unison with the body to create homeostasis. When the body's energetic system is out of balance, symptoms arise to ward off imbalance. Homeopathy, another energy force, works to reestablish the balance of the system by stimulating the defense mechanism and the natural healing abilities of the body.

Recovery is somewhat dependent on the degree of the body's degeneration. If severe, then regeneration is limited.

Basically, the intent is to discover the current energy pattern of the person's vital force. This includes symptoms, personality and lifestyle. Then, a remedy fitting the symptom and personality pattern can be given to provide a resonant reaction between the person's overall energy pattern and that of the homeopathic remedy. This reaction alters the existing pattern of disharmony, slowly bringing balance and recovery.

These are the basic principles of homeopathy as propounded by Hahnemann. They provide a foundation for further understanding. By no means are they complete, but they can help you in establishing a firm starting point.

Hahnemann's ideals bring dreams to reality. They become a part of every case and represent the natural flow of health, healing and balance.

Chapter Three

Casetaking: The Interview

During casetaking, people discuss their symptoms, personalities, family histories, traumas, surgeries and any other related aspects of their lives. We then begin to understand the core of their vital force. With this understanding we can understand the possible disharmony and how it has impacted or altered their life.

In Appendix B, there is an intake form that can be used for casetaking. At some point though, most homeopaths usually make up their own forms based on their specific needs and abilities.

The initial interview requires some preparation. First, select a private space that is clean, well-lighted, comfortable and quiet. Interruptions can be disturbing to both parties, especially when people are divulging painful events and emotions. These moments are unique and often difficult to recapture or repeat.

Second, after the person is seated, a brief explanation of the principles of homeopathy and the healing process can help in understanding the difference between homeopathy and standard medicine. It is a good time to establish a feeling of safety and trust. This initial description is patterned on a person's knowledge of homeopathy and the length of the description is dependent on that person's previous knowledge. I usually describe homeopathy in the following way:

"Homeopathy is a 200-year-old method of natural healing that stimulates your body to heal itself. By listening to various symptoms and asking questions, a pattern is established, giving a general overall picture of your life. Following this, a remedy is matched as closely as possible to create a cooperative energy between you and the remedy. Each remedy has its own picture, reflecting mental, emotional and physical components.

When a similar relationship matches between you and the remedy, the remedy acts to provide a spark to your vital force. This helps you to reestablish balance and eliminate symptoms.

All remedies are diluted to reduce side effects. Although, most symptom aggravations are slight, occasionally they can be extreme. These aggravations are a form of release to assist in strengthening your system and vital force rather than create further disharmony. Aggravations usually are of short duration, depending on sensitivities."

If there are any questions, address them after explaining homeopathy, so as not to interrupt the casetaking once it is started.

Next, get the person's name and address, phone number, age and occupation. Follow this by asking about the primary reason for the visit, the chief complaint. Allow the person to fully discuss current disharmonies or illnesses without interruption or questioning. During this time, observe the person's behavior, appearance and temperament while listening to symptoms. Take complete notes about symptoms, exclamations, examples and observations. Much is made of poor communication in our society, but in homeopathy, listening is crucial.

Through casetaking , many aspects are established, including restlessness, anxiety, skin coloring, ease of communication, eye contact or shyness. These observable symptoms are objective and valuable. If someone has freckles, it is obvious, and this, like almost everything else, is considered a symptom. Don't judge these symptoms or observations, for the responsibility of a homeopath is to gather information objectively and with compassion. Judgments create subjectivity not objectivity. A free and open mind is needed to assist in choosing the best remedy.

Casetaking: The Interview

After listening to the chief complaint and related symptoms, continue asking general open questions about any additional symptoms until they stop talking. Then wait for any final thoughts. During this entire time, there have been few, if any, specific questions from the homeopath.

Now, after having listened and observed, and after all symptoms have been described, the homeopath begins to ask questions in order to understand those symptoms. For each symptom described, specifically address the following:

1. When was the initial onset of your condition? How old were you?
2. How has the symptom changed over the years?
3. What is the frequency of reccurrence of the symptom?
4. What is the duration of the symptom. How long does it last?
5. How does it feel? What sensation does it have?
6. Does anything make it feel better or worse? (We call this a modality, i.e., if heat makes a person's joints feel better, then it can be found in the repertory and is valuable.)
7. Are there any concomitants? In other words, are there any other symptoms that arise with the original symptom? (A good example is a headache with irritability during menses.)

Upon completing these and any related questions, the essence of the person becomes clearer. The symptoms described reflect their personality along with any reactions to various stimuli.

Homeopaths often differ on the ways they do casetaking. Personal perceptions are meaningful. From this standpoint, a personal interviewing format is best.

One important thing to consider for the interview is etiology. This relates to the person's history and includes any family history. The interview lists all illnesses and predispositions, such as cancer, TB, children's maladies, emotional imbalances and organ problems. Specific questions relating to the person's past are significant. Get as much detail as possible to help understand any possible causes of present symptoms.

The following questions cover physical disharmonies, which is another important aspect of casetaking:

Appetite: Is it high or low, explaining why in detail?

Thirst: How much do they drink and what temperature?

Energy: Normal, high or low and what time of day is it low or high?

Food: Strong desires, aversions, and what disagrees, if anything?

Digestion: Any problems or irregular bowel movements? Gas?

Urine: Any odor, unusual frequency, incontinence, need to awaken in the middle of the night? Unusual color or blood?

Perspiration: Unusual odor or excessiveness? Head or foot sweats? Night sweats?

Skin: Dry, moles, warts, freckles, acne, eczema, itches?

Sleep: Insomnia, interrupted easily, hard to get to sleep (if so, why)? Restless? Position they first take upon going to sleep? Are they refreshed upon waking?

Dreams: Recurring or remembered? Feelings upon waking?

Menses: Any PMS, headaches, irritability, cravings, pains, unusual tendencies or related symptoms?

Sexual: Desires (high or low)? Fantasies? Masturbation? Frequency of sexual release?

Body Temperature: Usually more chilly or warm?

Seasons: Any strong preferences? Do they feel better or worse at certain times of the year? What is the feeling?

Sun/Moon: Better or worse in either? How?

Seashore/Mountains: Feel better or worse at either setting?

Wind: How does it effect them?

Allergies: To what? What effects or symptoms?

Exercise: Like or dislike it and how they feel afterward?

Other: Any other physicals that have not been mentioned or described? Get details?

Mental and emotional questions are often asked near the end of the interview. By this time, a person usually feels comfortable being questioned and they feel safe enough to be honest and open about their emotions. The mental area is considered one of the most important in homeopathy. It is within the psyche where you begin to grasp the deepest essence of the person.

Questions relating to emotions and emotional tendencies are frequently difficult for both parties. But, it is important to ask as many questions as necessary to fully comprehend the uniqueness and specific reactions of the person. Ultimately, homeopathy relates to certain emotional aspects of the person rather than just one symptom or pathology.

Emotions relate to feelings and energy. Mental disharmonies describe thought processes. Each is unique and significant to an overall presentation of the person's totality. Mental and emotional tendencies are given priority over physical symptoms. Emotions are energy in motion. When they are blocked or in excess, it says a great deal about the person's behavior.

Specific questions addressed in casetaking help in delving more deeply into a person's core emotions. Each emotion or mental aspect is important, and although tedious at times, should not be overlooked. Emotional components are listed alphabetically, and not necessarily in order of value. Additional emotional issues can be added if appropriate.

Anger: Is it expressed and how? Frequency of expression? At whom is it expressed? How long have they been angry? Any specific causes? Do they yell, scream, or get violent?

Anxiety: Do they worry? About what specifically? Frequency? About others, about the future, their health, about money? Where in the body is it felt?

Company: Do they prefer to be alone or with people? Which is stronger? Is solitude very important?

Consolation: How do they feel being consoled? Enjoy it or not?

Sympathy: Are they sympathetic? To what specifically? Do they take up causes? How do they feel about animals?

Excitable: How do they react to stimuli? Frequency? What is the most typical cause of it?

Fears: Describe in detail, even those of childhood or the past?

Concentration: Any difficulties? Any cause or injury? Forgetful? Apathy? Mental confusion? Trouble with words or mistakes in speaking? Ability to focus?

Grief: Loss of loved one or pet? Long-term impact and feeling it brings up upon discussion? How recent?

Impatience: What is the cause? How frequent? Give examples.

Irritability: Cause and frequency? How long does it last? Any food relationship or allergy? Does sleep deprivation affect them?

Critical: Of what and in what manner? Judgmental of self or others? How is it expressed? Any sarcasm?

Jealousy: What triggers it and how frequently? Envy? Suspicious or distrustful?

Guilt: For how long and about what?

Reproach: Is there self-blame or blame of others? How is it expressed or felt? Is there screaming or violence?

Yielding: Do they avoid conflict at all costs or are they prone to be more assertive or aggressive?

Moods: Are there quick swings or are they even? Highs or lows? Any known causes?

Restlessness: Can they relax? Do they always need to be active and moving (this is often observable)? Fingers, hands, feet?

Order: Is it important? Describe their room or office? How does clutter feel? How organized or sloppy? Do they save things?

Depression: How long and what cause? How is it manifested and are there related physical symptoms? Frequency and duration? Any suicidal tendencies? Any intent or past attempts?

Sensitivity: To what specifically? Noises? Odors? Light? emotions of others? How do they generally react? Intuitive? Are they oversensitive?

Weeping: Do they cry? At what and how easily? With music? Pains of others? Do they cry alone or in front of others? Do they cry telling their symptoms? Do they sigh telling symptoms?

Most symptoms have been described by this point, yet there may some the person has forgotten or does not want to talk about during the first interview. If you think this is true, ask questions without pressuring the person, to see if other symptoms are mentioned. These small bits of information can prove beneficial in understanding deeper disharmonies. Casetaking is now complete. It usually takes between one and two hours, but this time diminishes with experience.

Remember, do not ask leading questions, as yes and no answers may eliminate a deeper understanding of the person's disharmony. Ask general questions that allow detailed responses. Keep responses on track, especially when someone starts discussing unrelated events. Some people like to discuss their families rather than themselves, so gently bring them back to their purpose and their symptoms.

A sample casetaking may help you understand the process. This case will be used throughout the remainder of the book to show each different aspect of the homeopathic process.

A 41-year-old male suffers from asthma, which occurred following vaccinations before a trip to India some two years ago. Breathing is difficult especially after exercise, inhaling dust, cigarette smoke, or being in a warm room. It also comes on during sleep if there is no ventilation. The breathing problems and related symptoms are the chief complaint. Before the vaccinations, he had none of the above difficulties, although his father smoked a great deal as he was growing up. He has never smoked cigarettes. There is no family history of asthma, cancer or TB.

Observable symptoms include a neat appearance, athletic build but not overweight, some freckles, ridged fingernails, restlessness and an inability to sit still during the interview; he was always shifting position. He has clear skin, good coloring and he seems emotionally intense. Some observations can only be considered assumptions until further questioning provides clarity and validation.

To the best of his memory, the only major family illnesses, were diabetes and some arthritis. He personally had gonorrhea and was given antibiotics at an earlier age, without any long-term ill effects. He has no food allergies, but does get headaches either from tension, eating chocolate or reading without his glasses. He said that he had several concussions as a child, which could partly be the cause of the headaches. Nothing reduces the headache pain except a hot shower or a good night's sleep.

Food desires are varied, but he specifically likes sweets, pasta, pizza, cheese, chips and salsa, salads, fruit and veggies. He is a vegetarian, eating no meat, chicken or fish. He dislikes slimy foods and fish. He has trouble with sweets and cheeses. With sweets he gets headaches and gas. He gets a runny nose when eating cheese, especially just after eating it and again the next morning.

Digestion is normal, except for the gas, which he has had most of his life. He has occasional head sweats and ongoing foot sweats. He considers himself more chilly than warm, but is worse in a stuffy or warm room. He loves the sun, is affected by the moon (irritability) and enjoys both the seashore and the mountains. The wind is very annoying and makes him grouchy.

Emotionally, he gets angry easily and has most of his life if things don't go right (perfectionist?); he worries about money and his family (wife of seven years and three children);

he prefers being alone and but is fine with consolation. He has a slight fear of snakes, but no other obvious fears. Grief has not been a major part of his life, nor has guilt.

He is self-critical and judgmental of others, which includes blaming others for his own inadequacies. He is aggressive by nature, fastidiousness, controlling and dominating. He mentioned that his father is negative and he looks at life in much the same way.

These symptoms provide the picture of a man suffering from respiratory problems, anger, control issues and negativity. He also has a history of suppressed venereal disease, which could be the underlying cause of his current disharmony.

The analysis is presented in Chapter Five. In reviewing the case as presented, the core elements begin to surface. Take some time to visualize this person, to understand him and where his greatest disharmony lies. This is always addressed first, especially when it is life-threatening.

By looking at the whole person, certain symptoms become more prominent, along with the lifelong tendencies. Symptoms alone do not give a true picture, yet when combined with other observations, a distinct profile begins to emerge.

After completing the casetaking, symptoms are analyzed, reviewed and repertorized. After that time-consuming process, a materia medica is researched to determine which remedy fits the totality.

Homeopathic casetaking is unique to western medicine. It encompasses symptoms, pathology, personality, family history, injuries, emotions, desires, aversions, sleep patterns, body temperature, likes and dislikes, fears and anxieties. Many human conditions are touched upon in detail to find the relationship between remedy and symptoms. In this way, two unique, yet separate, energies come together to reestablish harmony and health: (1) the energy of the homeopathic remedy and (2) the person's unique energy. These two energies are joined in the dance of healing.

Homeopathic Vibrations

From casetaking to repertory, from the interview to finding the symptoms, from an empty canvas to the beginnings of color, the process continues to unfold and the mystery begins to unravel.

Chapter Four

Repertory: A Symptom Index

A repertory is an index of symptoms, taken from provings, clinical experiences and self-experimentation. The symptoms are called *rubrics*, with corresponding and related remedies systematically arranged for ease of use. There are hundreds of thousands of symptoms listed in a repertory, each of which lists remedies which have been proven to relate to specific disharmonies or symptoms.

During Hahnemann's lifetime, there were no repertories. He had his notes, successful case studies and his own materia medica. His findings were limited to 450 remedies. Today, we have over 2,500 proven remedies and many repertories. For decades, there existed one primary repertory, written by Dr. James Tyler Kent, M.D., in the early 1900's. It contained medical terminology of his time. In the past five years, the repertory has been updated and in one case, completely restructured.

Also, there are several software repertory programs available. For example, the following remedy list was taken from the rubric "confidence, want of self," in the Mind section of the computer version of the *Complete Repertory*, called *MacRepertory*:

MIND; CONFIDENCE; want of self, **Ambr, Anac**, <u>aur, bar-c</u>, <u>bry</u>, **Calc-f**, <u>chin, kali-c</u>, **Kali-p**, <u>lyc, med, nat-m, petr, ph-ac</u>, **Psor**, <u>puls</u>, **Sil**, sulph, tab, verat.

Note the bold identification in the above rubric. This represents the remedies that are of the highest degree and most effective for lack of confidence. The underlining represents the second degree and next highest effective remedies while the plain lettering reflects the least effective remedies, but still somewhat useful. The above is only a partial listing

41

of all the remedies under the rubric, but it gives you an idea of rubric and remedy relationship from a repertory.

Kent's version of the repertory is written in a way unique to his thinking, his times and his homeopathic experience. It is a compilation of the great homeopaths of his day in an attempt to consolidate symptoms into one book for easy reference. His intent was to supply a source for all homeopaths to use in locating remedies for their analysis.

His first chapter deals with mental and emotional symptoms from the word "Abandoned" to the last rubric titled "Wrong, everything seems." Kent felt that mental and emotional symptoms were the most important of a repertory. Interestingly enough, he considered the section on the Generalities to be the second most important for discovering the true core of disharmony. However, he placed this chapter last in his book.

After the Mind Chapter are the following sections, each of which deals with physical disharmonies and particular aspects of physiology. The information following each heading represents specific symptoms relating to those headings:

Vertigo: time of day, when, where and physical sensations.

Head: including hair, headaches, pains, sensations and injuries.

Eye: sensations, discharges, eruptions, irritations and pain.

Vision: blurred, astigmatisms, colors, effected by; loss of.

Ear: abscess, discharge, eruptions, itch, noises, pain and wax.

Hearing: loss of, impaired and illusions.

Nose: hayfever, discharges, types of discharges, dryness, nosebleeds, fullness, itching, obstruction, pain and smell.

Face: discoloration, expressions, eruptions, pain, heat and cold, wrinkles, ulcers, veins and swelling.

Mouth: abscesses, bleeding, discoloration, dryness, herpes, inflammation, odor, pain, tongue, salivation, speech, taste, swelling and tumors.

Teeth: decay, discoloration, pain, looseness, grinding and sensitivity.

Throat: choking, discoloration, dryness, enlargement, heat, inflammation, irritation, mucus, pain, swallowing, sensitive, tonsils, spasms and ulcers.

External throat: goitre, pains, stiffness, sensitivity and swellings.

Stomach: anxiety, appetite, food desires and aversions, constrictions, bloating, eructations, heartburn, heat, indigestion, nausea, pains, thirst and vomiting.

Abdomen: anxiety, liver, distention, flatus, spleen, hernia, pains, inflammation, tension and ulcers.

Rectum: constipation, diarrhea, hemorrhoids, bleeding, itch, pains, incontinence, prolapse and straining.

Stool: color, types, frequency and odor.

Urinary Organs:

Bladder: sensations, stones, inflammation, pains, retention, urging and urination.

Kidneys: inflammation, pains and suppressions.

Prostate: emissions, enlargement, inflammation and pain.

Urethra: constriction, discharge, bleeding, inflammation, itching, pains, sensations and swelling.

Urine: sensations, color, types, amounts, odor, sediment.

Genitalia:

Male: desires, aversions, atrophy, erections, herpes, eruptions, inflammations, testicles, itch, pains, discharges, sensitivities.

Female: miscarriage, bleeding, menses, desires, aversions, cancer, dryness, herpes, inflammation, itch, discharges, menses, menopause, pains, tumors, sterility.

Larynx and Trachea: constriction, croup, sensations, mucus, inflammation, irritation, dryness, pains, swelling, voice.

Respiration: anxious, arrested, asthmatic, difficult, impeded, irregular, sighing, snoring, wheezing.

Cough: time of day, types, sensations, aggravations, duration, croup, whooping.

Expectoration: types, color, difficult, odor, mucus, taste.

Chest: abscess, anxiety, heart, congestion, cancer, lungs, pains, mucus, eruptions, fluttering, bleeding, bronchitis, inflammation, breast milk, nodules, palpitations, ulcers.

Back: bifida, sensations, eruptions, curvature, inflammations, injuries, pains, stiffness, tension, weakness.

Extremities: arthritis, awkwardness, hands, fingers, arms, legs, feet, toes, knee, nails, sensations, frostbite, corns, joints, cramps, discoloration, eruptions, injuries, pains, lameness, heaviness, numbness, paralysis, restlessness, stiffness, swelling, trembling, ulcers, weakness.

Sleep: disturbed, dreams, position, restless, insomnia, yawn, unrefreshing.

Chill: time of day/year, sensations, exposure, internal, shivers, sides of the body.

Fever: sensations, time, alternating, cerebro-spinal, cough, dry, continuous, perspiration, intensity, rash, gastric, intermittent, septic, sun, zymotic.

Perspiration: time, causes, anxiety, types, exertion, odor, profuse, sleep, suppressed.

Skin: burning, itching, eruptions, herpes, shingles, hot/cold, discoloration, bruises, gangrene, freckles, inflammation, sensitive, sore, bites/stings, birthmarks, ulcers, warts, wrinkles.

Generalities: aggravations covering the entire body, including time of day/year, anemia, air, cancer, lack of vital heat, food, clothing, convulsions, faintness, VD, injuries, loss of fluids, lassitude and weakness, motion, obesity, pains, pulse, sensitiveness, standing/sitting, swelling, touch, varicose veins, wounds and wind.

As previously mentioned, Kent's work is somewhat outdated, yet the format is still being used by a majority of homeopaths. They continue to upgrade material with remedy additions and new rubrics on a regular basis. Two new ones to consider are *The Complete Repertory* by Roger Van Zandvoort and *Synthesis* by Dr. Frederik Schroyens.

A third repertory by Dr. Robin Murphy has altered the format by alphabetizing the sections, and by adding new rubrics and remedies. He has combined various symptoms into their pathology picture, such as chronic fatigue, candida and compulsive disorders. Others have used this alphabetical system, but not nearly as completely or as recently.

Probably the best way to understand the use of a repertory is by repertorizing a case. Using the asthma case described in the last chapter as our example, we discover that each symptom described can be located in a good repertory. At times though it does require interpretation or research to find those exact symptoms and relate them to repertory terms.

Usually the first step requires choosing the predominant symptoms, but in this instance, analysis is left for the following chapter.

A few random rubrics will serve to clarify the process. The chief complaint of the 41-year-old was asthma which occurred following the vaccinations necessary for his trip to India. His asthma became worse after exercise, worse with dust and smoke, and worse in a stuffy room during sleep.

Using *Kent's Repertory*, we find "asthma, coming on during sleep" in the Respiratory section on page 765. These are the listed remedies under that rubric:

Acon, Ars, Carb-v, Hep, Kali-c, Lach, meph, Nat-s, op, sep, Sulf.

Remember, the underlined remedies are in the second degree and not as strong as the bold type remedies, of which there are none in this instance.

To help understand the procedure for repertorization, write each of these remedies in a column down the left side of a piece of paper, at the top of which is labeled the symptom, i.e., Asthma, sleep. < is the symbol for worse and > is the symbol for better.

Continuing in the Respiratory section, look up Difficult on page 769 and find two rubrics, "dust, as from" and "exertion, after". The remedies in the dust rubric are:

Ars, aur-m, bell, <u>Brom, Calc</u>, cycl, <u>Hep</u>, ip, nux-v, phos, **Sil**, sulf. (Note that there are two remedies in bold here.)

Start another column with the symptom < *dust* at the top and list the remedies down the column. Do the same for the rubric < *exertion*, listing all the remedies in the column.

It should look something like this:

Asthma, sleep;	Difficult Resp. <dust;	Difficult Resp. <exertion
Acon	Ars	Apis
Ars	aur-m	Ars
Carb-v	bell	Ars-i
Hep	Brom	Aur-m
Kali-c	Calc	brom
Lach	cycl	Calc
meph	Hep	Camph
Nat-s	ip	Carb-v
op	nux-v	Ip
sep	phos	Lach
Sulf	Sil	Nat-s
Sulf	Sulf	Nux-v
		Sil

All the remedies have not been listed nor placed in the degree of their strength, as organization of rubrics and remedies are the only aspects currently being considered. It becomes a matter of simple addition when the symptoms have been listed, i.e.. adding up the remedies for the highest total. The highest number does not always reflect the best remedy, for that comes with the analysis of the person in conjunction with their symptoms.

In searching for the rubric, *worse since vaccination*, look to the Generalities section under vaccination, page 1410 where there are nine remedies listed, including several previously listed in the above rubrics: <u>Ars</u>, **Sil**, **Sulf**, hep.

Repertory: A Symptom Index

This gives you an idea of the lengthly effort needed to repertorize an entire case, as only four rubrics have been examined and there are over 30 remedies listed so far. The whole case has about 50 separate symptoms described by the patient, so analysis in choosing specific predominant symptoms becomes very important. The analysis begins to eliminate certain rubrics and consolidate others, allowing for a concentrated effort toward the most similar remedy.

To assist in further understanding how a repertorization search works, read the repertory sections, specific rubrics, unusual terms and review casetaking procedures. By becoming more familiar with the material, the process becomes easier. Symptoms can be located and remedies eliminated as one grows more comfortable with a repertory and its index of symptoms.

A few additional notes about a repertory that can be of aid when reviewing symptoms and studying its rubrics:

There is a specific arrangement in each section, beginning with the time of day, proceeding to conditions of the body in alphabetical order, then various pains with their locality and character.

Symptoms are generally those that cause aggravation to the entirety, unless the rubric specifically denotes that the symptom is ameliorated. For instance, in the Mind section on page 12 under Company, the rubric is: amel., when alone. This means that they feel better when they are alone.

According to Kent's theories, the Mind and Generalities sections are the two most important ones. The former relates to the mental and emotional aspects while the later reflects the body as a whole. On page 1358 of Kent's Repertory, the rubric *Exertion, physical*, means that any physical exertion aggravates the whole body. They feel worse with exercise.

Food is broken down into two separate sections. The first is in the Stomach section and consists of desires and aversions. The second is in the Generalities section and is consistent with which foods aggravate or have ill effects on the whole body.

There is a word index in the back of the book which can be valuable for finding the various symptoms described. It is also important to get a good medical dictionary.

Modalities are described in almost every section and relate to heat/cold, motion/rest, position and hours of the day or night. The modalities are excellent directional signals to the correct remedy as they usually are unique to the individual.

The repertory covers both chronic (of long duration), and acute (self-limiting and of short duration), cases. Both require good casetaking for the best results.

Familiarize yourself with the repertory by just picking it up and reading through it on a regular basis, then research the words that are unfamiliar.

There are two areas with large pain sections: Head and Extremities. Take time to review these sections to help with headaches and extremity problems.

A repertory is a useful tool for finding remedies. It is also an important tool in understanding the principles of homeopathy. Do not minimize the initial effort necessary to become familiar with this material as it will serve you well in the future.

Much like a directional detour sign which provides a better route, a repertory directs us to specific symptoms and remedies. Ultimately, the more we understand specific symptoms, the better the result.

You have taken the case and a repertory has given you some direction with several remedies. But, it is the analysis that provides the detective work for elimination of symptoms.

Chapter Five

Case Analysis: Unraveling the Mystery

Case analysis involves examining the person's present-ing symptoms and deciding which are important and which are not. This is especially necessary when the person has described over 50 varying symptoms and perhaps 20 different modalities within those symptoms.

Many approaches have been successful and most homeo-paths develop a system that feels comfortable, personal and effective. The purposes of analysis are twofold. First, is the discovery of the similar remedy for the given circumstances. Second, and just as important, is the completion of casetaking with an understanding of the person as a whole.

The second purpose is of value because there are times when the best-suited remedy is not effective, despite the time taken to evaluate a case. At this point, it requires more than the totality of symptoms, as the person's vital force may manifest specific symptoms which create underlying causes. These causal factors, when clearly perceived, will assist in understanding why a remedy was ineffective.

Why does a well-chosen remedy not work? Several reasons come to mind, including misreading the individual. Also, layers of disharmony can block a true response. Perhaps symptoms were not given proper weight in the first evalu-ation, or the core essence of the case was not reached or perceived adequately.

Each case is gleaned through the person's own words, body language and observations as well as questions asked by the homeopath. It is easy to misread someone if a case is not taken properly or completely. Perhaps questions were not direct enough or the homeopath did not delve deeply enough into emotional disharmonies. If there is any uncertainty about the case or something appears incomplete, thorough questioning can uncover the answer.

Layers of disharmony are developed over a lifetime. Starting from the trauma of birth we unintentionally alter our body's natural ability to regenerate by taking drugs, medicine, smoking, environmental exposure, etc. Additional layers such as stress, auto accidents, surgeries, sensitivities, foods, chemicals, drugs, medications, vaccinations and the environment, affect a person. These effects alter the normal energetic patterns we are born with, and create layers of disharmony.

Each layer produces its own pattern, often requiring specific attention in order to be eliminated or balanced. If, on the other hand, we find that a specific thread runs through the entire case, despite the layers, then we have a grasp of the essence. For instance, in the case of the 41-year-old man with asthma, there are several threads running throughout his life that shows a deeper disharmony, both physically and emotionally. This also reflects certain susceptibilities.

If a layer has so altered the energetic patterns of his entire being, then that layer must often be addressed before the best remedy can be found or be effective. If a car accident has created headaches and other physical or mental problems, then symptoms from the accident and those after the accident must be evaluated first, especially if those symptoms strongly affect the person's current lifestyle.

The weight given various symptoms relate to their intensity and life-threatening tendencies. Asthma can cause major disharmony if untreated so it is given more weight than a rash or a digestive problem. Each symptom is evaluated according to how it affects a person, how limiting it is and how long it has been a part of their life. Also, a person's spontaneous description of their symptoms, without prompting, is given stronger credence than those that require questioning, simply because of the natural flow of expression. Attaching a weight to each symptom is a key to understanding which rubrics to choose when repertorizing. The effect of a hurricane is much greater than a gentle blowing breeze.

Symptom weight is based on the most limiting symptoms in the presenting picture. For instance, with a flu where there is difficult respiration, fever, diarrhea, headache, a cough that is exhausting and nasal discharges, the first order of priority is the respiration. If we don't breathe, we die! Next, comes the loss of body fluids because this is significant when excessive, and can be very depleting. The cough, fever and headache are less severe. The symptoms may change, leaving a prescriber to evaluate based on the most limiting or debilitating symptoms. Common sense tells us which are the most limiting symptoms. How to choose which symptoms, can be determined by the presenting state of the person's disharmony.

To understand the core essence of a person, not only is good casetaking necessary, but getting them to freely discuss their personality traits is also important. If the person is shy, unaware of family history or old symptoms, emotionally closed, private, or just a person who likes to please, it is difficult to get to the core of the case. Questioning alone will not work in this instance, so the issue of openness and honesty is best emphasized at the outset. Still, someone may want to hide certain aspects of their personality because of past shame or fear. Again, reassure them before the process begins so as to eliminate this possibility. It may take several visits before a person will feel comfortable enough to discuss certain issues

If you have done everything possible to overcome these obstacles, and enough information is still not available for a good evaluation, then stop the interview and have the person return at a later date. Perhaps writing down past memories of childhood, talking to relatives or checking medical histories will be of value. Pressure to evaluate and discuss symptoms serves neither party.

Let's return to the previously described asthma case as this may assist you in further understanding the analysis process. Remember, the chief complaint is asthma. Since it is the most limiting symptom described, repertorization covers each specific modality along with the associated cause—vaccination. The remedy selection is one that must include the asthma complaint, not only because it is the primary symptom, but because of its unique limitation.

The next rubric to add is from the Mind section, "anger over mistakes," which has only three remedies on page 2 of *Kent's Repertory*. Too few choices are limiting with respect to remedy selection and in a situation of that nature, looking to the larger general rubric, "anger" expands the choices without eliminating remedies too soon. Why choose the anger rubric? Because, it represents lifelong emotional disharmonies and may relate to the liver, an organ of vital importance in the body.

Two of the observed symptoms—restlessness and intensity—provide objectivity while providing a deeper perspective into the core of the person. "Restlessness while sitting" on page 74 of Kent has 11 remedies, and as this may be too limiting, we can include the rubric "internal restlessness" to fill it out and give a broader range from which to choose.

Intensity is not a rubric and here is where we can fully begin to understand the complications that arise when symptoms are not specifically described in the Repertory. When a person discusses a symptom that is not mentioned in the Repertory, specific questions about feelings and meanings are important. Perhaps it is a feeling about deeper emotions that need to be understood or explained.

In the asthma case, intensity is an observed symptom so the question can be posed directly whether he feels as if he is normally an intense individual. If yes, delve further. If no, describe your observations and ask for an explanation of his feelings surrounding that observation. If no further clarity is obtained, then it may be necessary for you to disregard the observation. In the Repertory, intensity could mean "absorbed," "anxious," "serious," or may relate to "concentration," all of which are rubrics.

If it appears that one of the above rubrics does relate to intensity, get clear descriptions of the specifics, especially for any anxiety symptoms, as this is a large rubric.

Returning to the emotional components of the asthma case, he described himself as critical, negative, blaming, controlling and fastidious.

The rubric for the symptom *critical* is "censorious" and is relatively large. Although it does require some extra effort to write each remedy in a column, learning is important and will aid in understanding the complete process. The closest rubric to negative is "contrary" as there is no rubric for pessimism in *Kent's Repertory*. Several of the newer repertories do have this rubric, along with the term "negative." Just as before, write all the remedies in a single column with the symptom at the top of the column.

The symptom described as blaming is found in the rubric "reproach" and covers both "self-reproach" and "reproach of others." In Kent, controlling is located under the rubric "dictatorial", which also means demanding. Continue with the columns and the headings with each particular symptom discussed.

The rubric for fastidious is on page 42 of *Kents' Repertory* listing only two remedies, and although several additional remedies have been added to the newer Repertory versions, this one is too small for analysis and will not be used for now. On page 16 is a larger rubric, "Conscientious about trifles," which has some relationship to fastidiousness, but this is not the description given and must also be avoided unless additional clarification warrants its use.

There are several other emotional symptoms, but the ones described provide a good representation of the symptom picture. Covering the totality of the case does not always mean using every symptom described. It is more of the choice of symptoms which most reflect the core essence.

Recalling some of the physical symptoms of the asthma case, he mentioned he is chilly, feels worse in a stuffy room, is generally worse during a full moon, is irritable in the wind and is aggravated from cheese and sweets. These rubrics can be located in the Generalities section of *Kent's Repertory*.

Chilliness is found in the section entitled "Heat, lack of vital" and each remedy mentioned is a chilly type remedy. There is not a perfect rubric for feeling worse in a stuffy room, so this symptom is interpreted to mean "desires open air" on page 1343 of Kent. It could also mean worse on "becoming heated," under "Heated" in the Generalities section, but desires open air fits best in this situation. Aggravation from the full moon is found under "Moonlight aggravates" and is too small of a rubric to be used for evaluation or analysis.

Irritability or aggravation from wind is a large rubric on page 1422 of *Kent's Repertory* and will be added to the symptom and remedy columns. Next, are the food aggravations: cheese and sweets. Cheese is a dairy product, so the rubric "worse dairy" can be combined with the smaller cheese rubric to create a larger remedy selection. The rubric, "sweets aggravate" can be found on page 1364.

In the Generalities section is where the rubric "Vaccination, ailments after" can be located. Some homeopaths consider that when venereal disease acquired earlier in life has been suppressed, it should be released. This is found under the section "Gonorrhea, suppressed" on page 1365. It will not need to be added to the columns since once the most suited remedy is found, a release of preexisting symptoms arises naturally.

The remainder of the symptoms can be used to confirm final remedy choices, but at this point are unnecessary for analysis. Adding all the symptoms together, there are 6 asthma rubrics and 16 mental and general rubrics, for a total of 22 rubrics and columns. As mentioned earlier, the first remedy to be selected must be in the asthma rubrics and also in several of the 16 other rubrics described. Rarely will a remedy be in all of the rubrics. And on occasion, the highest scoring remedy is not the best-suited one because it does not fit the person's essence. Add up the 22 columns and get the top five remedies—the remedies listed the most times from all columns.

Through experience, additional means of elimination are combined into the analysis process. Perhaps only 10 rubrics are necessary to determine an effective remedy. For now, it is not recommended that any of the following be pursued until the basic methods are mastered. The foundation of analysis comes from established principles which provide the basis for all further procedures. Early shortcuts only create habits that may delay effective treatment. Additional analytical tools include:

Common and Unusual symptoms: Common symptoms are usually disregarded as they do not reflect anything unique or indicative of the essence, such as a cold. On the other hand, peculiar or unusual symptoms are extremely important and effective in discovering specific remedies. Often, these peculiar symptoms have few remedies listed, but are so unique as to mandate inclusion in the final picture. A good example is "desires to be alone when urinating." Quite unique and it has only has a few remedies.

Symptom weight: Generally the Mentals and Generals are given the highest importance and value. But if a particular or physical symptom can be evaluated as significant, then it is given greater weight in the remedy selection. Examples would be asthma, bleeding, or heart problems.

Modalities: These are unique symptoms relating to what makes a person feel better or worse. They assist in finding the extraordinary relationship a person has with their illness. Modalities can be useful in every component of the analysis, including mentals, generals and particulars. If there are specific modalities for common symptoms that aid in creating a uniqueness, then they can be used with those also. A predominant modality can also provide an insight into the person's basic nature. For instance, the modality—worse in sunlight or worse in winter—shows a unique expression of how a person is affected at the deepest levels. A modality is the soul of a symptom and very important. Choose the most dominant ones to help you during analysis.

Concomitants: This reflects a combination of symptoms that occur together. A good example is "runny nose with each stool." Not only are there two symptoms here, but they represent a unique symptom picture. There is only one remedy listed in this rubric—Thuja. So consider it to be valuable in defining the final remedy choice. By combining separate symptoms that occur at the same time, such as headache with menses, a larger picture is created where one did not previously exist. Also, a more complete picture is established combining rubrics and increasing the number of available remedies.

Description: A person may emphasize certain symptoms with body language or tone of voice. Generally, it is more important how the symptom is described rather than what is described. Look for the redness of the face or the irritability when asked a question, the contempt in the voice or even a tendency to avoid direct responses to questions. This will assist you in discovering the essence of the personality, which is especially true for mental symptoms.

Latest symptoms: The most recent symptoms reflect a current picture of the vital force and are used more frequently than older ones. Often, existing symptoms contain indicators for past disharmonies. Older symptoms may not be as distinct or clear as present ones, and the most similar remedy, the Simillimum, will release older, suppressed disharmonies. There are occasions where current presenting symptoms may not involve older imbalances, but by working with existing pictures and previous symptoms, the first remedy will become more obvious.

Chief symptoms: The first symptom mentioned, provides a point of departure as it applies to many remedies, such as asthma. Do not use the pathology alone, as this precludes modalities and the essence of the person. Determine which symptoms affect the person strongly, which are the most limiting in their life and use these to bring about change.

Three particulars: When the person describes several similar symptoms, like burning in the stomach, burning with breathing and burning upon swallowing, combine these symptoms into a single rubric, "Pains, burning" in the Generalities section. This pulls together three different rubrics while reducing the possible remedy selections.

Etiology: This reflects the underlying cause of the disharmony. Often, the cause is unknown upon first glance, but questioning can uncover the event or time when certain changes occurred and any relationship to a specific trauma. Cause is a key aspect to analysis and cannot be overlooked. An example would be headaches during menses or ovulation, the cause of which is probably hormonal imbalance.

Elimination: Getting to a reasonable number of rubrics requires an understanding of symptoms, remedies and the person. Ten rubrics should be enough to reach a conclusion about remedy selection and still include the personal nature. The asthma case had 22 rubrics, after eliminating unnecessary ones. That number can be further reduced to include those which reflect the totality, the essence, the causes, the emotions and the pathology:

1. Cause of the asthma: vaccinations.
2. Restlessness is a deep disharmony and is observed rather than stated by the person.
3. Chilly is in Generalities and reflects the whole person.
4. Suppressed veneral disease may be the cause of deeper disharmony and this symptom gives some understanding of the person.
5. Anxiety about money. Why this worry and few others? Because it is an important symptom for him.
6. Fastidiousness was mentioned and observed, providing an insight into his core from two separate perspectives. This is so because it is a unique symptom component.

7. Anger, because it is a lifelong emotion.

8. Controlling may have an underlying cause like insecurity. This is confirmed by his being critical, self-demanding and blaming. Even though he did not mention that self-esteem was an issue, it obviously cannot be overlooked.

9. His desire for sweets and cheese can be used to confirm remedies.

10. Aggravation from wind is an objective symptom.

The remainder of the rubrics or symptoms are not disregarded, but will not be necessary for this analysis. Totality does not always mean repertorizing all the symptoms described by the person. It means using rubrics which can be used to provide an accurate portrait of the case's essence.

Remedies: The selection of a single remedy is the final process in analysis. To reach this point, only four or five of the top remedies are considered. Frequently, the final remedy is not in every rubric chosen, but is found in the predominant ones. After adding the numbers in each column and narrowing the search to four or five final remedies, each remedy is reviewed fully in the materia medica to determine the closest Simillimum. Materia medica serves to clarify which remedy will be of greatest value in the moment.

The top five to consider and review are:

1. Thuja
2. Silica
3. Sulphur
4. Arsenicum Album
5. Medorrhinum

A remedy which does not relate to the person, their symptoms or their essence may create a proving. As long as there is some relationship between the person and the remedy, remedy provings rarely arise. The five listed above all have various points in their favor and some which don't relate to the person, such as the general heat of Sulphur. Which would you choose as the first remedy?

Chapter Six

Materia Medica: The Key

Books on materia medica represent hundreds of years of compilation, experience, provings, clinical evaluations and healings. The information within these unique volumes reflect complete remedy portraits from mental, emotional and physical disharmonies. There are over 2500 remedies, with regular additions and updates.

Some of the remedies are quite specific and somewhat limited in their presentation, while others are highly detailed. These full, rich and complete remedies cover numerous maladies and are called *polycrests*. The following books are a must for the beginning homeopath and will help you better understand the remedies.

Boericke's Materia Medica with Repertory: This work includes the vast majority of remedies, and although somewhat outdated in its terminology, is helpful with the less detailed remedies.

J. H. Clark's Dictionary of Materia Medica: Like Boericke, this covers almost all remedies, but also includes specific characteristics and stories of the remedies along with symptoms and provings.

Hering's Condensed Materia Medica: Ten volumes reduced to a single volume, while the strongest symptoms remain intact for each one.

Kent's Lectures on Homeopathic Materia Medica: An excellent resource for 180 remedies with insights into Dr. Kent's unique approach and his work.

Gibson's Studies of Homeopathic Remedies: Written within the last three decades, this work covers 120 remedies including the source for each of them along with clinical notes and general appearance.

Morrison's Desktop Guide: An outstanding modern Materia Medica that covers over 200 remedies, with updated terminology, comparisons and clinical aspects.

Murphy's Lotus Materia Medica: Currently being revised to include over 1,200 remedies, this book is modern, insightful and incorporates remedy folklore.

Materia medica is the final source for evaluation and remedy selection. Rarely will a determination be made without reviewing materia medica to get a "feel" for the person in connection with the chosen remedy. The term *materia medica* means medical material which has been compiled from symptom pictures along with numerous other sources.

In Chapter 5, repertorization of the unique aspects of the asthma case was completed. The conclusion was that several remedies closely resembled the symptom totality. Those particuler remedies each have their own signature. Whichever one relates to the essence of the presenting symptoms, will be the one that is most effective for aiding recovery. This is the point where materia medica proves invaluable, as the remedies can be reviewed for making final decisions. In alphabetical order, the remedies that were the strongest after repertorizing were:

Arsenicum Album: This remedy has a strong relationship to many aspects of the case; there is chilliness, worse since being vaccinated, tendency to be fastidious, lacking self-esteem, controlling and restlessness. Also, it is an effective asthma remedy.

Silica: It has many similar components to Arsenicum, but without the anger or as much anxiety. Silica tends to be yeilding rather than controlling. They also lack stamina.

Sulphur: They are too warm-blooded and do not have the anxiety reflected in the case.

Nux Vomica: Similar to Arsenicum in many ways, but they are not worse after being vaccinated and do not have the anxiety or restlessness.

Thuja: They do not have the restlessness, controlling tendencies or anxiety, but are worse after vaccinations and have suppressed veneral disease, along with being fastidious.

Lycopodium: This remedy has most of the mentals described, but is not very strong in the generalities or physicals.

The best-suited selection comes from reading about each remedy in more than one materia medica. This helps you find out which ones seem to fit the person and not just their symptoms. By narrowing the remedy selection to five or six remedies, the final choice becomes easier, especially after repeated review. Occasionally, a remedy will be a perfect fit, but more often, the remedy relates strongly to the most limiting aspects of the case and becomes very effective.

With all the excellent books on materia medica, it is important to buy several for your homeopathic library. Rather than provide complete sketches of the major polycrests, the following information supplies some of the key aspects of 62 specific remedies. As mentioned above, a remedy is best studied in its entirety by reviewing it from more than one materia medica. In that way, a complete picture of every component of the remedy along with its relationship to the physical, emotional and mental essence becomes clearer.

Morrison's Desktop Guide, covers 156 remedies in detail and provides an overall picture for each. As an example, the remedy *Nux Vomica* is a large polycrest which a large segment of society may need at some point in their lives. With his permission, the following is Morrison's review for Nux:

"The typical Nux Vomica patient is readily recognized by almost all homeopaths and is in fact one of the most commonly prescribed remedies.

Work: The popular concept of "type A personality" describes the typical Nux Vomica patient very well. The Nux Vomica patient is impatient, competitive and ambitious. The major focus of his life is on work and achievement. He is confident and even arrogant. The patient is compulsive with his work and in all aspects of his life, even to the point of fastidious cleanliness and ordering of his house or office.

Anger: People of such a focused nature often have strongly aggressive personalities, and this is very characteristic of the Nux Vomica patient. The patient can be irritable, first only sporadically but as he becomes more pathological the irritability becomes anger, then rage, then frank violence. In the usual case, however, the patient is irritable mainly from impediments to his ambitions. He becomes infuriated at the slowness and inefficiency of his co-workers, of waitresses, cashiers, etc. Even an inanimate object can anger the patient: he may tear his shirt if the buttons don't come out easily; he breaks the phone if he gets a busy signal on an important call. He may have long standing, unresolved anger towards his parents or others. In advanced states, the patient develops increasingly violent behavior patterns which may even end in criminal behavior.

Competition: In almost all aspects of his life the Nux Vomica patient is competitive. When he plays cards he must win; when he jogs, he must jog faster than the others on the track; when he drives, he cannot bear the idea that the person in the next lane may get ahead of him, so he switches lanes to always be in the fast lane even if that requires forcing himself into the path of another car. He wants to try everything and is not overly cautious about things he may explore. Any type of stimulant - coffee, alcohol, amphetamines, even cocaine will attract this patient. He may also be hedonistic in sexual matters. The Nux Vomica patient fears and avoids marriage, not out of fear of responsibility as in Lycopodium but from fear of the loss of freedom or fear of being humiliated in marriage.

Collapse: It is easy to understand that the patient described could be subject to collapse states from over-work or abuse of substances or from indulgence and excess. Nux Vomica is one of the best remedies for patients in collapsed states, not only for the collapse itself but to help him to be more moderate in his behavior in the future.

Physical: On the physical plane, Nux Vomica pathology centers largely on the gastrointestinal tract. Since so many of the symptoms of Nux Vomica are related to its heavy strychnine content, it should come as no surprise that spasm and cramping are very prominent. Additionally the nervous system is often disturbed.

Children: The Nux Vomica child is irritable and often affected with gastrointestinal problems such as colic or colitis. As school age comes the child is competitive about his grades and sports far beyond the norm. He is a terrible loser. The parents may say that the child can under no circumstances admit that he is at fault or that he has made a mistake. Jealousy of the other siblings or toward other gifted children at school is often a problem. In adolescence the child may develop strongly bitter feelings towards his parents, especially the same-sex parent. It can be astonishing to find how rudely such a child can speak towards his parent in such cases. These children are very concerned about fair-play both towards themselves and others and can seem very idealistic. Many Nux Vomica children exhibit strong fears, especially fear of the dark.

Mind

IRRITABLE, IMPATIENT, AMBITIOUS AND DRIVEN PATIENTS.

EASILY OFFENDED. Anger from contradiction.

Tendency to break things from anger and frustration.

Premenstrual irritability.

IMPATIENT: HATES WAITING IN LINES OR IN TRAFFIC.

COMPETITIVE. WORKAHOLIC. COMPULSIVE.

Fastidious, especially angry if objects not in their proper place.

Fear: Marriage. Humiliation. Dark (especially in children).

Failure.

Substance abuse. Alcoholism. Delirium tremens.

Weeping from anger. Weeping before menses.

Aversion to tight clothing - in a hurry to take off watches, ring, tie.

Great sensitivity to stimulation - light, noise, odors, etc.

General

<Chilly and worse from cold and from cold, dry wind.> CHILLS, RIGOR FROM MOVING UNDER HIS BLANKET (during fever).

<Generally better from warmth and warm applications.

<Collapse and fatigue states from over-work.

General aggravation from alcoholic drinks or from abuse of alcohol.

Breakdown from substance abuse. Simple "hangover".

General aggravation from eating.

Convulsions, worse anger, worse touch.

Faintness, worse odors, worse labor.

Cerebral accidents with paresis, expressive aphasia, convulsion.

General aggravation from dry weather.

General aggravation from suppressed hemorrhoids (peptic ulcer).

Acute's

Influenza or other febrile conditions with high fever and violent chills and rigors which are worse from every movement which stirs the air under the covers.

Cystitis with nearly constant urging, relieved for moments only on passing small quantities of urine and relieved by warm applications or warm bathing.

Gastritis with pains from alcohol abuse or from over-eating.

Acute colic - kidney stones, cholecystitis - with cramping pains better from heat, worse touch.

Head

Headache and migraine, worse noise, worse light, worse mental activity or vexation, worse before menses.

Photophobia.

Allergy and hay fever, even hay asthma.

SNEEZING AND CORYZA IN MORNING ON WAKING OR ON RISING.
Fluent coryza in the morning but obstructed at night.
Coryza worse in open air.
Bruxism.
Gastro-intestinal
Craving: <Spicy. Fat. Alcohol. Coffee. Tobacco. Any stimulant.
Peptic ulcers in workaholic patients. Gastritis from alcohol abuse.
Hepatitis, either infectious or alcoholic.
Nausea and vomiting, worse anger, worse alcohol, worse menstrual colic or other abdominal pains, worse smoke.
<Stomach pains, worse anger, worse tight clothes, better warmth, warm applications or warm drinks.
<Cramping or sharp pains in abdomen, worse after eating, worse cold, better warmth or warm drinks, better stool.
<Infants with colic and angry arching of the back.
Rectum
CONSTIPATION WITH CONSTANT, INEFFECTUAL URGING FOR STOOL; small amounts are passed which temporarily relieves the urging only to return moments later.
Constipation in children with hard, painful stool; the child fears going for stool.
Diarrhea alternating with constipation; constant urging for stool but passes small amounts. Diarrhea, worse cold, worse alcohol.
Urging for stool during urination.
Hernia, inguinal or umbilical.
Hemorrhoids; pains better warmth, better after stool.
Urinary and Sexual Organs
CYSTITIS WITH CONSTANT URGING FOR SMALL AMOUNTS, BETTER WARM BATHING.
Painful urinary retention.
Sex drive increased; promiscuity.
Kidney stones; renal colic.

Pyelonephritis.
Dysmenorrhea with urge for stool before or during the flow.
Uterine or rectal spasm during sexual orgasm.
Chest
Cough, worse morning, or morning in bed.
Asthma, often worse exertion, worse night, worse 3 or 4 AM, worse cold, worse in the morning.
Angina pectoris.
Palpitations from coffee, from excitement.
Extremities
<Back pain, worse night in bed, worse turning in bed, must rise to turn, worse during fever, worse during urge for stool.
Fibrositis, worse cold, better warmth.
Cramps and contractures of muscles.
Twitching, tics, tremor and muscle spasms anywhere in the body.
Sleep
INSOMNIA, WAKES ESPECIALLY 3 OR 4 AM AND CANNOT SLEEP DUE TO THOUGHTS ABOUT WORK or how to accomplish tasks.
Sleepiness during day, worse eating, worse when sitting, worse watching TV.
Clinical
Alcoholism. Allergy. Angina. Arrhythmia. Arthritis. Asthma. Behavior disorder. Cerebral accidents. Chemical sensitivity. Chronic fatigue syndrome. Colds. Colic. Constipation. Crohn's disease. Cystitis. Endometriosis. Fibrositis. Headache. Hemorrhoid. Hypertension.Inflammatory bowel disease. Influenza. Insomnia. Irritable bowel syndrome. Kidney stones. Low back pain. Lupus. Migraine. Multiple Sclerosis. Neuralgia. Peptic ulcer. Premenstrual syndrome. Prostatitis. Pyelonephritis. Rectal fissure. Sciatica. Ulcerative colitis.
Complimentary
Sulph. Kali-C. Phos. Sep. Staph.
Comparisons

Med: Extremes of behavior, workaholic, irritable, allergy, peptic ulcer, craves fat, alcohol and spicy, urinary symptoms, etc.

Lil-T: Intense irritability, dysmenorrhea, ineffectual urging.

Cham: Anger, over-sensitive to stimulation, colic.

Sep: Irritable, thin, sensitive to noise, premenstrual syndrome, constipation, abuse of drugs, cystitis, etc.

Sulph: Ambitious, arrogant, craving fat and alcohol, hemorrhoids, colitis, insomnia, etc.

Aur: Workaholic, haughty, irritable, insomnia, craving alcohol.

Calc: Workaholic, breakdown from over-work, chilly, constipation.

Ign: Easily offended, ambitious, cramps and spasms, rectal pathology, back pains."

As you can see, the review is comprehensive and complete. It covers many aspects of a person, including various pathologies, and the essence of the remedy. Each polycrest has a picture as complete as this one, yet they also have their own core or specific uniqueness.

After getting such a wonderful picture of Nux Vomica from Dr. Morrison, it is easier to understand the complexity of each polycrest. What follows are 62 remedies in a short form covering more of the uniqueness, rather than specific comprehensive aspects. Each remedy is best-studied in its entirety. Studying the essence alone does not provide the flavor, it just supplies a starting point for basic understanding.

ACONITE: worse after cold, wet weather; anxiety and fears; shock; panic attacks; early or sudden onset of illness; restlessness.

ALUMINA: anxiety from being hurried; dullness; mental slowness; dryness of all membranes; constipation; disorientation; dizziness; itchiness of the skin without eruptions.

ANACARDIUM: low self-esteem; abusive; cursing; depression; fears and delusions; controlling; violent and angry;

brain fatigue; most symptoms are better from eating; strong sexual desires.

APIS: redness, itching, swelling; busy; thirstless; right-sided ailments; worse from heat applications.

ARGENTUM NITRICUM: anxiety and panic attacks; impulsive; feelings of abandonment; open and excitable; warm blooded; worse eating sweets, but craves them; gastrointestinal problems; left sided ailments; many phobias.

ARNICA: trauma and injuries; concussions; bruises; irritability; prefers be alone; relief of pains; refuses doctors help.

ARSENICUM ALBUM: anxiety; restlessness; avarice; compulsive; fearful; depressed; skin disharmonies; chilly; controlling without spontaneity; right-sided ailments; worse around midnight; asthma; thirst for small sips; burning sensations.

AURUM: severe suicidal depression; serious; self-condemnation; guilt and abandonment issues; worse cloudy weather; intense; worse with pain; anger with remorse; moans during sleep.

BARYTA CARBONICA: slowness in mental development; immature behavior; low self-esteem; shy and yielding; anxious and nervous; chronic tonsillitis; blank facial expression.

BELLADONNA: early onset with redness, heat, flushing of the face and fever; delirium; anger intense with hitting, biting; migraines; thirstless; strep and sore throats.

BRYONIA: worse with any movement/motion; irritability; prefers solitude; fear of business or financial failure; dry mucus membranes and dry colon; intense thirst; warm blooded; joint problems.

CALCAREA CARBONICA: overly responsible; bone problems; fear of heights; fear of going insane; overwhelmed; slow development as a child; stubborn; overweight; slow metabolism; head sweats; milk allergy.

CALCAREA PHOSPHORICA: complains about everything; loves change and travel; dissatisfied; sensitive; craves smoked foods; state of weakness; grief with sighing; slow development.

CANTHARIS: urinary tract infections; burning sensations; strong sexual desires; incontinence; violent emotions.

CARBO VEGETABILIS: intense irritability; gastrointestinal problems; negative; prostration and weakness; coma; indifference; coldness; air hunger.

CARCINOSIN: intense, sympathetic, passionate; family history of cancer; fastidious; craves chocolate and spicy food; moles on back; strong libido; loves animals; low energy from 3 to 6 p.m.; loves travel.

CAUSTICUM: idealistic and rebellious; sympathetic; serious; very sensitive to suffering of others; grief; joint and TMJ problems; warts; compulsive; desires smoked foods; chilly; incontinence.

CHAMOMILLA: peevish when ill; intense irritability; excessive sensitivity to pains; infant desires to be carried; one cheek red, other pale; colic; ear infections; teething problems; worse travel.

CHINA OFFICINALIS: internal sensitivity; introverted; taciturn; gastrointestinal disharmonies; worse loss of fluids; anemia; colitis; worse touch; periodicity of complaints; fear of animals.

CONIUM: emotional flatness or indifference; paralysis; cancer; hardness of glands; tumors; fixed ideas; fogginess of the brain.

CUPRUM: spasms and convulsions; appears emotionally closed; sensation as if suffocating; flat facial expression; seizures; rigid; intense emotions suppressed.

FERRUM METALLICUM: anemia; desires raw meat; overweight; face flushes easily; very sensitive to noise; strong willed; better walking slowly; general weakness and fatigue; demanding.

GELSEMIUM: fatigue; heaviness of the eyelids; brain fatigue; stage fright; weakness of will; cowardly; indifference; forgetful; tremble with anticipation; depressed; thirstless; chilly; headaches; diarrhea.

GRAPHITES: slowness with poor concentration; skin abnormalities; irritable; anxious; herpes; indecisive; many self-doubts; fastidious; overweight tendencies; offensive sweats; restlessness; photophobia.

HEPAR SULPHURIS: anger when security is threatened; irritable; worse any draft of air; sensitive; chilly; infections and abscesses; intense and hurried; rarely cheerful; abusive· overreact to pains.

HYOSCYAMUS: paranoia; jealous with violent outbursts; intense sexual desires; worse with touch; hyperactive child; shameless; defiant; delusions; talkative; fear of dogs; wild gestures.

IGNACIA: acute grief or worse since grief; romantic/idealistic; aggravation from consolation; prefers be alone; stress is better after eating; better with exercise; sighing; disappointed love.

IODUM: very warm; thyroid disfunctions; very restless and busy; compulsive; talkative and anxious; impulsive; intense appetite; anger; avoids company; discontent and destructive; general fears.

KALI BICHROMICUM: sinus disharmonies/headaches; strong sense of right and wrong; thick, yellow, ropy discharges; rigid and proper; self-occupied; suppresses emotional aspects of personality.

KALI CARBONICUM: righteousness and strong sense of duty; mind rules the emotions; fear of losing control; rigid; asthma; possessive; conservative; quarrelsome; self-reproach; worse 2 to 5 a.m.

LACHESIS: left-sided complaints; loquacity; suspicious; jealous; sarcastic; opinionated and can be fanatical; warm blooded; all types of menstrual disharmonies; intense personality; vindictive; active mind; drug and alcohol addictions; low self-esteem.

LEDUM: prefers solitude; hatred for self and others; joint problems; worse heat, although chilly; worse movement or motion; irritable; insect bites, lockjaw, or injuries with bruising; puncture wounds.

LYCOPODIUM: poor self-confidence; anger and irritability; liver and kidney disharmonies; fears and anxieties; hyperactive children; right-sided ailments; low energy 4 to 8 p.m.; anticipatory anxiety; tendency to dominate or control; opinionated; avoids responsibility; digestive problems; generally chilly but prefers open air and worse warmth.

MAGNESIA MURIATICA: yielding; aversion to confrontations; feels anxious at night; very responsible; noises annoy; composed, with suppressed inner anger; depression; unrefreshing sleep.

MEDORRHINUM: nasal discharges; cruel and aggressive behavior; an extremist; "sex, drugs and rock 'n roll"; self-centered and love danger; obsessive/compulsive; history of VD; hurried; intense passions; bites fingernails; overwhelmed by impulses; night person; loves sea.

MERCURIUS: strong reaction to temperature changes; emotionally closed; stammering speech; conservative; anxious with destructive ideas; paranoia; facade; worse at night; excess saliva; night sweats; serious appearance; metallic taste in mouth; gum infections.

NATRUM CARBONICUM: very sensitive; craves potatoes; inner turmoil and depression with appearance of cheerfulness; prefers solitude; emotionally closed; sweet and selfless; delicate; poor digestion; worse heat and sun; sadness; milk allergies; sympathetic.

NATRUM MURIATICUM: fear of being hurt; closed emotionally from past grief; very sensitive; critical; perfectionist; romantic; strong desire for solitude; serious and controlled;

introverted; depression; generally worse from being in the sun or heat; hayfever; herpes.

NATRUM SULPHURICUM: head injuries and concussions; suicidal depression; very responsible and serious; warm blooded; feels better after a bowel movement; emotionally closed; asthma; possible past history of venereal disease; sensitive; practical, with business focus.

NITRICUM ACIDUM: generally negative person; self-discontent and anger; curses; restless; hypersensitive; selfish; anxieties about health and death; vindictive; chilly; pains come and go suddenly.

NUX VOMICA: Type "A" personality; ambitious; meticulous; hypersensitive, with tendency to overreact; liver and bowel remedy; driven to excess; addictive personality; sensitive nervous system; intense irritation from wind; chilly; insomnia with waking at 3 a.m.

PETROLEUM: skin disharmonies of all types, with dryness; quick temper; motion sickness; herpes; offensive perspiration; unable to make decisions; chilly, worse in winter; increased hunger.

PHOSPHORICUM ACIDUM: dullness and slowness; apathy; feels overwhelmed with grief and emotions; intense fatigue and loss of energy; yielding; desires refreshing fruits; dehydration; chilly.

PHOSPHORUS: expressive and extroverted; prefers consolation and company; impressionable and very sensitive; many fears and anxieties; affectionate; chilly, yet likes cold drinks; craves spicy, salty and sweets; sympathetic; intuitive; nosebleeds.

PLATINUM: primarily a female remedy; haughty to the extreme; is worse with touch; idealistic; dwells on the past; feels abandoned; dislikes children; insolent and rude; pretentious; strong libido.

PLUMBUM: taciturn; sad; shy; selfish; difficulty in expressing themself; indifference; illness slow in development; very chilly; pains tend to radiate; neurological disorders.

Materia Medica: The Key

PSORINUM: skin disfunction of all types; periodicity; pessimist; tend to despair with hopelessness; anxiety and fear, especially of poverty; very chilly; low energy; feels forsaken/lost; dirty skin.

PULSATILLA: warm blooded; capricious mood swings; PMS; mild and dependent nature; female remedy; abandonment issues; desires consolation; weepy; digestive and sinus (thick yellow/green mucus) problems; worse heat and craves fresh air; thirstless with dryness.

RHUS TOXICODENDRON: great internal restlessness; obsessive tendencies; skin and joint remedy; feels better stretching and with motion; withhold affections/feelings; apprehensive at night; timid; herpes with burning and itching; worse cold/damp.

RUTA: affects tendons and fibrous tissues; distrustful; startles easily; argumentative; stiffness/pain; strains/sprains; eyestrain; related headaches; worse motion or lying on painful side.

SEPIA: indifference and desire to be alone; impatience; irritability; low sexual desires; chilly; grief and depression; PMS/menopause; bearing down sensations; leucorrhea; taciturn and negative; herpes.

SILICA: yeilding; timid and bashful; emotionally dependent; low self-esteem; stubborn; chilly; conscientious about details; constipation; slow development; weakness; perspires easily; recurring infections.

SPIGELIA: left sided ailments; serious; responsible; violent pains; migraines; grief; worse tobacco smoke; anxiety of pointed objects; pinworms; combination heart and eye symptoms; chilly; worse touch.

SPONGIA: fear of suffocation; heart ailments; increased anxiety; dry mucus membranes; dry, barking, croupy cough; easily frightened; thyroid disharmonies; respiratory conditions; weakness.

STAPHYSAGRIA: sweet, yielding person; suppressed emotions; very sensitive; emotionally dependent; fear of losing control; possible history of sexual abuse or humiliation;

strong sexual history; grief; suppressed anger; low self-confidence; worse after a nap; mild.

STRAMONIUM: violent tendencies; etiology from a fright; impulsive rage; wild behavior; night terror; desires company and light; intense thirst; flushed face; excitable; stammers; convulsions; promiscuous; hyperactive children; could be mild, gentle and very sensitive.

SULPHUR: idealistic and philosophical; self-contained; indolent; warm blooded; burning sensations; desires spicy foods; appearance is not important; collects things; opinionated; desires open air; itch; offensive discharges; offended by other's body odor; aversion to bath.

SYPHILINUM: compulsive tendencies; worse at night; very chilly; alcoholic; excess saliva; fear of disease/germs or going insane; nails are distorted; anxious; indifferent; worse hot or cold extremes.

THUJA: low self-confidence; emotionally closed and hard to get to know; secretive; fastidious; hurried; herpes and suppressed venereal disease; ailments after vaccinations; urine stream is forked; runny nose with stool; chilly; left sided ailments; irritable; warts; oily skin.

TUBERCULINUM: desires change and travel; feels unfulfilled; can be mean; compulsive; chilly; respiratory disharmonies; milk and cat allergies; hyperactive children; romantic longings; desires smoked foods; excess perspiration at night; itch, better with heat.

VERATRUM ALBUM: self-righteous and haughty; thinking more than feeling; precocious child; hyperactive child; ambitious; deceitful; very chilly; abusive spouse; critical; jealous; restlessness; religious mania; excessive cold sweats; inappropriate kissing or hugging.

ZINCUM: hypersensitive and overstimulated; impulsive movements; restlessness; always complaining; mentally overwhelmed and fatigued; worse when drinking wine or alcohol; superstitious; chilly; affected by noises; feels better after eating.

Materia Medica: The Key

These remedies are only a small portion of the 2,500 remedies available. However, 70 to 80 percent of all cases will be well-served by using one of the above remedies. Studying complete details of each polycrest creates an understanding about the depth and strength of the remedy. And in doing so, you get a feel of its essence and grasp its identity. Do not rely on these brief remedy descriptions to determine effectiveness in a case.

Many of these 62 remedies are the most frequently prescribed ones, but they are also the most often listed in the repertories. This provides a strong sense of their usefulness for casetaking and healing. There are other valuable remedies, especially some of the less detailed ones, so avoid shortcuts in prescribing or in understanding materia medica.

Studying and understanding remedies is a long-term process, filled with questions and doubts. Many remedies have similar traits and symptoms, but each has some unique component to set it apart from the others. These are the aspects that give a deeper comprehension of its essence and help establish a better grasp of the whole remedy.

When one looks at a special painting from a master such as Van Gogh, one finds similar tendencies and attitudes in the various works, but each painting has it's own style and uniqueness. Remedies are similar in this respect, but only by looking into the deeper essence can you find the true energy flavor that will resonate with the unique energy flavor of the person. Perhaps it is like tasting rum-flavored raisins, one could never discover the actual taste by appearance alone.

Next, are acute illnesses, covering various problems that arise from germs and bacteria. In working with homeopathy and acute disharmonies, it is important to note whether or not the illness is life-threatening before trying to use the described remedies. Caution and common sense go together in dealing with health problems. Call a health care provider if there are any questions or doubts about the person's symptoms or the intensity of those symptoms.

Chapter Seven

Acute Disharmonies: The Short Term

An acute illness is one which is self-limiting, meaning that it has a life span of approximately seven to ten days. Without any assistance, it usually expires on its own. There are occasions where an acute illness serves a valid purpose by releasing accumulations of toxins while allowing the system to become stronger and more vital. In that situation, the body can find its own balance in its own time without prescribing a remedy.

Just as often, the illness feels as if it is overwhelming and quite debilitating. This can cause a state of collapse from its intensity. Homeopathy is not used for every symptom that arises, as these symptoms are the body's messages of disharmony. A fever is a message that there is an infection and body heat is a means of disarming or eliminating the infection without interference. By allowing the system to function as much as possible without outside influences, the body finds a way of recovery and, what is most important, a way of reestablishing the vital force.

A tree that has been blown over from the wind can be replanted and recover fully without additional support. It just required deeper planting to support itself and continue to grow. Our body is much the same, if given the opportunity to find its own healing path.

When symptoms become intense or fear arises at the onset, consider the cause and choose a remedy related to the totality to accelerate the healing process.

The following presentation covers various acute illnesses along with some proven remedies. These brief symptoms will help you in using homeopathy for short-term acute cases and can be helpful in some emergencies. Obviously, if there is a crisis or critical situation, common sense dictates that proper

medical treatment be obtained. On the other hand, homeopathic remedies are excellent for shock and emergencies
while a person is being transported to the hospital or health
care provider. If you have time to evaluate the symptoms
along with the person involved, it is wise to do a complete
work-up.

Accidents

ABRASIONS/CUTS:

  Arnica for trauma of all types and bleeding, even coma.
  Calendula for antiseptic use, either internal or external.
  Hypericum for injury to nerve endings or incisions.
  Ledum helps heal puncture and penetration wounds.

BURNS:

  Cantharis reduces pain and promotes healing process.
  Urtica Urns for first- and second-degree burns.
  Hypericum reduces pain when nerve endings are involved
  such as spine, fingers and teeth.
  Belladonna for fever, flushing of the face and delirium.

BITES:

  Ledum for all types of bites with coldness around area.
  Hypericum when pain seems excessive for the wound.
  Belladonna for dog and snake bites.
  Lachesis for snake bites or with flushes of heat .

BRUISES:

  Arnica for bruises or muscle injuries.
  Bellis for trauma, contusions and soreness.
  Hamamelis helps with internal bleeding and bruising.
  Ruta for stiffness in muscles and tendons from bruising.

BLEEDING:

  Phosphorus for all types of hemorrhaging.
  Ferrum Phosphoricum helps coagulate the blood.
  Lachesis when blood is dark and area is blue.

Ipecacuanha for gushing, bright red blood with nausea.

HEAD INJURIES:

Arnica for all types; Conscious or unconscious.
Cicuta for dilated pupils, muscle spasms and stiffness.
Gelsemium for occipital pain and heaviness of the eyes.
Hypericum for numbness, tingling and seizures.

SHOCK:

Aconite after a sudden fright or fearful situation.
Arnica after an injury or trauma, causing shock.
Carbo Vegetabilis for fainting, coldness and difficulty breathing.
Veratrum Album when skin and perspiration is very cold.

WHIP LASH:

Bryonia when any movement is painful.
Causticum when neck muscles and tendons contract.
Hypericum if nerves and a tingling sensation is involved.
Rhus Tox for injuries that are better with motion and heat.

Allergies

ANAPHYLACTIC SHOCK:

Apis for constriction, inflammation, swelling, hives, redness of the skin and soreness; Worse with heat.
Urtica Urns for eruptions, itching, blotches and burning; Heat with a stinging sensation.
Consider: *Arsenicum Album; Natrum Mur; Rhus Tox.*

TO ANIMALS:

Arsenicum Album for respiratory-related reactions.
Allium Cepa for clear, burning nasal discharge with runny eyes.
Euphrasia for profuse, burning discharge from eyes.
Natrum Mur for egg white-like discharge; Cannot smell.
Consider: *Sabadilla; Nux Vomica; Tuberculinum; Sulphur.*

TO CHEMICALS:

Arsenicum when there is a burning sensation afterward.
Coffea for excitability of the mind and nervousness.
Mercurius when you feel worse at night with excess sweat.
Nitric Acid for the oversensitive, depressed and negative types.
Consider: *Nux Vomica; Phosphorus; Sulphur; Psorinum.*

TO DUST:

Arsenicum Album when respiration/wheezing is involved.
Bromium when there is a feeling of suffocation and coldness.
Hepar for heart palpitations and anxious wheezing.
Consider: *Silica; Ipecachauna; Pothos.*

TO FOODS:

Beans: Bryonia; Lycopodium; Petroleum; Calcarea Carb.
Bread: Bryonia; Lycopodium; Natrum Mur; Pulsatilla; Sepia.
Cheese: Arsenicum; Nux Vomica; Phosphorus; Sepia.
Coffee: Cantheris; Causticum; Chamomilla; Nux Vomica.
Fruit: Arsenicum; Bryonia; China; Colocynthis; Pulsatilla.
Meat: Arsenicum; Calcarea; China; Ferrum; Kali Carb.
Milk: Calcarea; China; Magnesium Mur; Natrum Carb; Sepia.
Onions: Lycopodium; Thuja; Sulphur; Ignacia; Pulsatilla.
Potatoes: Aluminum; Bryonia; Silica; Sepia; Pulsatilla.
Salt: Carbo Veg; Natrum Mur; Drosera; Phosphorus; Silica.
Starches: Berberis; Lycopodium; Natrum Mur; Lachesis.
Sugar: Argentricum Nit; Lycopodium; Sulphur; Phosphorus.
Vegetables: Aluminum; Bryonia; Kali Carb; Natrum Sulf.
Wheat: Allium Cepa; Lycopodium; Natrum Mur; Pulsatilla.

Acute Disharmonies: The Short Term

HAY FEVER:

Arsenicum Iod. for profuse watery discharges and tickling.
Wyethia for itching of the palate and dry mucus membranes.
Arundo has burning and itch in nostrils with sneezing.
Arum for sneezing and tickling sensations; Congestion.
Consider: *Arsenicum; Allium Cepa; Sabadilla; Euphrasia.*

INSECT BITES:

Ledum for any puncture wound with coldness around the wound
Apis for red, hot, swollen skin that is worse with heat.
Hypericum for tingling sensations or numbness.
Urtica Urns for hives, itching, redness and worse with heat.
Consider: *Arsenicum; Belladonna; Thuja; Lachesis.*

POISON IVY:

Bryonia has swelling, heat, dryness, thirst and is irritable.
Anacardium for intense itch with swelling and redness.
Croton Tig. for painful scratching and pustules; Intense.
Graphites for a watery discharge from the reaction.
Consider: *Clematis; Rhus Tox; Sepia; Sanguianaria.*

TO SMOKE:

Euphrasia for burning in the eyes and nasal discharge.
Ignacia when breathing is affected; person feels annoyed.
Sepia for nausea and exhaustion with any left-sidedness.
Spigelia for dryness, tickling and constriction in throat.
Consider: *Nux Vomica; Natrum Mur; Causticum; Sulphur.*

Children's Remedies

COLIC:

Chamomilla desires to be carried, is irritable and angry.
Colocynthis for a bloated stomach with intense pains.

Dioscorea for arching back with cramping pains and gas.
Magnesium Phos when a child feels better bending double with the cramps.

CHICKEN POX:

Aconite for the first stages of the outbreak.
Antimonium Crudum overheated and angry.
Rhus Tox for restless, intense itch with swollen glands.
Sulphur for a burning itch, and is worse in heat and sweat.

COLDS:

Aconite for sudden onset from cold, dry winds.
Belladonna for early stage with fever, redness and thirst.
Kali Bic when discharge is thick, yellow/green and ropy.
Pulsatilla for thick yellow mucus and clinging to parent.
Consider: *Allium Cepa; Euphrasia; Hepar; Nux Vomica.*

COUGHS:

Barking: Aconite; Belladonna; Drosera; Spongia.
Croupy: Aconite; Hepar Sulf; Spongia; Lachesis; Phos.
Dry: Belladonna; Bryonia; Drosera; Natrum Mur; Rumex.
Hacking: Allium Cepa; Arsenicum; Drosera; Phosphorus.
Rattling: Antimonium Tart; Causticum; Dulcamura; Ipec.
Violent: Belladonna; Causticum; Cuprum; Lachesis; Phos.
Whooping: Antimonium Tart; Carbo Veg; Cuprum; Drosera.

DIARRHEA:

Arsenicum for a watery, burning stool with nausea.
China for a painless stool containing undigested food.
Podophyllum for frequent, gushing stool that is smelly.
Rheum for sour smelling stool resulting from teething.
Consider: *Nux Vomica; Sulphur; Silica; Rhus Tox.*

EARACHE:

Aconite for the early stages with cold symptoms.
Chamomilla when pain and irritability arise together.
Hepar for smelly discharges; is worse when cold.

Pulsatilla for congestion with redness and discharge.
Consider: *Lycopodium; Silica; Mercurius; Belladonna.*

FEVERS:

Aconite for sudden onset with anxiety, heat and dryness.
Belladonna for flushed face, burning heat and delirium.
Gelsemium for shivering, heat, drowsiness and no sweat.
Mercurius for excess saliva; Heat alternates with chills.
Consider: *Natrum Mur; Nux Vomica; Pulsatilla; Sulphur.*

INFLUENZA:

Oscillicoccinum for the earliest stages, within 24 hours.
Baptisia for prostration, muscle soreness and stomach.
Eupatorium when there is deep bone ache and debility.
Gelsemium for drowsiness, aches, chills and exhaustion.
Consider: *Arsenicum; Bryonia; Rhus Tox; Nux Vomica.*

INDIGESTION:

China when gas arises after eating fruit; Bloated.
Ignacia from any type of emotional upset.
Lycopodium for gas and bloating made worse from eating.
Nux Vomica from overindulgence of food or drink.
Consider: *Argentricum Nit; Pulsatilla; Carbo Veg; Sulphur.*

MEASLES:

Aconite is excellent for early stages.
Belladonna for fever; is used in the early stages.
Bryonia for cough, fever, dryness and intense thirst.
Pulsatilla is restless and desires attention; No thirst.
Consider: *Gelsemium; Apis; Euphrasia; Phosphorus.*

MUMPS:

Belladonna for swelling, fever, heat and redness.
Jaborandi for redness, swollen glands and excess saliva.
Mercurius for painful swelling, fever and profuse sweat.
Rhus Tox for swelling with fever; Better with heat.
Consider: *Aconite; Apis; Lachesis; Phytolacca; Pulsatilla.*

RASH (Diaper):

Apis for red, sore, shiny and hot skin; Worse with heat.
Petroleum for dry, red, itching and cracked skin.
Rhus Tox is better with hot bath; Skin itches, flakes and burns.
Sulphuric Acid for blotchy, red skin; Worse with heat.
Consider: *Sulphur; Graphites; Mezereum; Urtica Urns.*

SORE THROAT:

Aconite for heat and fever from dry cold winds
Belladonna is the first choice with heat and redness.
Causticum for burning, soreness, rawness and tightness.
Phytolacca for congestion, redness and very painful.
Consider: *Apis; Hepar; Lachesis; Mercurius; Gelsemium.*

TEETHING:

Belladonna for pain, fever, shrieking, restless and flushed.
Calcarea Phos for slow, difficult dentition.
Chamomilla for intense pain, irritability and hot cheeks.
Pulsatilla for clinginess; painful dentition. Better in fresh air.
Consider: *Coffea; Silica; Kreosotum; Rheum; Phytolacca.*

Headaches

MIGRAINE:

Bryonia for a pressing sensation with thirst; Worse with motion.
Gelsemium for dull, droopy mind fog; Blurred vision.
Glonoine for throbbing pain, heaviness and irritability.
Melilotus for bursting pain with red face and nausea.
Sanguinaria for right-sided pain that radiates to eye; Worse in the a.m.
Consider: *Belladonna; Iris; Coffea; Apis; Nux Vomica; Spigelia.*

TENSION:

Argentum Nit for an enlarged head feeling with impulsiveness.

Ignacia when you feel worse from any emotional stress or anxiety.

Natrum Mur feels like pounding hammers; Worse 10:00 a.m.; Throbs.

Phosphoric Acid when apathetic; Worse from loss of fluids or emotions.

Zincum when exhausted, nervous and restless; Noise sensitive.

Consider: *Coffea; Gelsemium; China; Nux Vomica; Thuja; Phos.*

HORMONAL:

Cyclamen for a flickering sensation; Worse in open air and when chilled.

Kreosotum for menstrual headaches with irritability.

Lachesis for deep pain, coming in waves; Left-sided with burning.

Sepia feels as if there is a band around the head; Left side; Sad.

Pulsatilla for when you feel weepy, sad, thirstless and are sweating; Better in open air.

Consider: *Lycopodium; Natrum Mur; Belladonna; Lac Caninum.*

SICK:

Cocculus for motion sickness, loss of sleep or noise.

Chelidonium for liver-related and right-sided with drowsiness.

Nux Vomica for overindulgence of any kind.

Picric Acid for mental strain, fatigue or travel.

Consider: *Iris; Ipecachauna; Sulphur; Arsenicum A; Sanguinaria.*

Homeopathic Vibrations

SINUS:

Dulcamara for changes in barometric pressure; Worse in damp air.
Euphrasia for burning sensation in the eyes with tearing.
Kali Bic for burning sensation at root of nose; Pain in one area; Sinusitis.
Mercurius for excess saliva, bad breath and metallic taste.
Consider: *Calcarea Sulf; Hepar; Nux Vomica; Thuja; Natrum Mur.*

PERIODIC:

Arsenicum for one specific time of day with burning; Better with heat.
China worse from loss of fluids or malaria; Liver ailments.
Nitric Acid for burning nasal discharge; Worse with pressure.
Silica for radiating pains, head sweats, worse drafts, chills.
Consider: *Natrum Mur; Sanguinaria; Sepia; Lachesis; Ignacia.*

Sports Injuries

BROKEN BONES/FRACTURES:

Arnica for the earliest stage of trauma or injury.
Bryonia when pain is intense from any type of motion.
Calcarea Phos helps in formation of callus in fractures.
Symphytum helps bones to properly knit after being set.
Consider: *Hypericum; Rhus Tox; Ruta; Silica; Calcarea.*

DISLOCATIONS:

Carbo Animalis for diminished strength and tendon contraction.
Kali Nitricum for numbness, heaviness and weakness of limbs.
Calcarea when the problem is chronic and fails to heal.
Ruta when tendons are involved, especially wrist and ankle.

Consider: *Arnica; Natrum Carb; Rhus Tox; Lycopodium; Bryonia.*

PULLED HAMSTRING:

Bellis for soreness, stiffness, coldness and bruising.

Ambra-G for drawing pain; limb seems shortened; Tingling.

Causticum for hardness of tendons and contractions; Cramps.

Ledum for swelling and stiffness; Better with ice.

Consider: *Arnica; Ruta; Rhus Tox; Bryonia; Sulphuric Acid.*

HIP POINTERS:

Aesculus for radiating pain that is worse upon standing.

Calcarea Phos for stiffness; Worse with motion or air drafts.

Rhus Tox if stretching reduces pain; Better with heat.

Ruta for lameness and stiffness; Better when lying down.

Consider: *Arnica; Bellis; Hamamelis; Symphytum; Bryonia.*

SPRAINS/STRAINS:

Bryonia when worse from any movement; Wants to be alone.

Bellis for stiffness with a bruised sensation.

Asafoetida for hysteria with bone pains and inflammation.

Millefolium for tearing pains from overexertion; Irritable.

Consider: *Arnica (first); Rhus Tox; Ruta; Ledum.*

Travel

CONSTIPATION:

Alumina has no desire for stool or may strain; Straining; Worse with travel.

Bryonia for dark, dry, hard stool; Very thirsty for cold water.

Nux Vomica when bloated and irritable; Never feels fully vacated.

Silica for ineffectual urging; Hard stool which pulls back in.

Consider: *Plumbum; Sulphur; Opium; Aloe; Sepia; Nitric Acid.*

DIARRHEA:

Aconite after cold, dry wind or fright.

Arsenicum for prostration, vomiting, restlessness and anxiety.

China after eating fruit or a summer chill; Painless; Fever.

Colocynthis for intense colicky pains; Better with pressure.

Consider: *Nux Vomica; Veratrum A; Podophyllum; Aloe; Sulphur.*

INDIGESTION:

Anacardium for heartburn two hours after eating; Pain/fullness.

Carbo V for offensive gas, bloating, pain and internal heat.

Lycopodium when bloated with pain; Better after passing gas.

Nux Vomica is worse after overeating; Gas, bloating and cramping.

Consider: *Arsenicum; Bryonia; China; Pulsatilla; Sulphur; Hepar.*

INFLUENZA/COLD:

Ferrum Phos for the earliest stages without clear symptoms.

Baptisia for prostration, cramps, nausea and confusion.

Gelsemium when achy, chilled, weak and anxious; Heavy eyelids.

Eupatorium Perf. for deep bone aches with chills and headache.

Consider: *Arsenicum; Bryonia; Nux Vomica; Rhus Tox; Hepar.*

JET LAG:

Cocculus when lack of sleep causes irritability and fatigue.

Gelsemium for heavy eyes, headache, weakness and tired limbs.

Argentricum Nit for fear and panic while flying; Anxious.

Arnica for being cramped in a seat for a long period.

Consider: *Rescue Remedy; Phos Acid; Zincum; Sulphuric Acid.*

MOTION SICKNESS:

Borax for nausea or vomiting; worse with downward motion.

Cocculus for queasiness; Worse with the thought of food.

Nux Vomica for nausea, headache and chills; No desire for food.

Tabacum when chilled, giddy and sweating; Worse with tobacco smoke.

Consider: *Rhus Tox; Petroleum; Ipecachauna.*

SLEEPLESSNESS:

Arsenicum for restlessness, anxiety, fatigue and irritability.

Coffea when nervous, anxious, hypersensitive and mentally active.

Ignacia when worse from emotional stress or grief.

Nux Vomica when worse from overeating, alcohol or mental strain.

Consider: *Aconite; Lycopodium; Pulsatilla; Arnica.*

STRESS:

Natrum Mur for long-term emotional ill effects and solitude.

Nux Vomica when there is mental stress and overstimulation.

Passiflora when overworked, worried, restless and exhausted.

Valerian when oversensitive, irritable, nervous and changeable.

Consider: *Zincum; Arsenicum; Argent Nit; Ignacia; Sepia.*

Women's Ailments

CYSTITIS:

Apis for burning, stinging and soreness when urinating.

Cantharis for intense urging, burning which is passed by drops.

Equisetum for bladder fullness, severe pain and frequent urge.

Lycopodium for low back pains, straining and retention.

Consider: *Aconite; Belladonna; Lachesis; Sepia; Pulsatilla.*

DISCHARGES:

Black: China; Kreosotum; Rhus Tox; Secale.

Bloody: Calcarea Sulf; China; Cocculus; Nitric Acid; Sepia.

Burning: Calcarea; Borax; Kreosotum; Pulsatilla; Sulphur.

Green: Carbo V: Kali Bic; Mercurious; Natrum Mur; Sepia.

Itching: Calcarea; China; Mercurious; Sepia; Kreosotum; Zincum.

Milky: Calcarea; Kali Mur; Sepia; Silica; Pulsatilla; Lachesis.

Offensive: Kali Arsenicum; Kreosotum; Mercurious; Nux Vomica.

Profuse: Calcarea; Graphites; Sepia; Silica; Stannum; Thuja.

Thick: Arsenicum; Calcarea; Kali Bic; Natrum Carb; Thuja; Zinc.

Thin: Graphites; Nitric acid; Pulsatilla; Sulphur; Silica; Sepia.

White: Borax; Graphites; Natrum Mur; Sepia; Nux Vomica; Puls.

Yellow: Arsenicum; Calcarea; Chamomilla; Hydrastis; Puls.

GENITAL HERPES:

Natrum Mur for tingling sensations; Worse in sun or under stress.

Petroleum for sensations of moisture with crusting and itch.

Sepia for itching, worse at folds of skin and in spring; Odor.

Thuja for eruptions on covered parts only; Sensitive to touch.
Consider: *Rhus Tox; Alnus; Medorrhinum; Lachesis; Dulcamura.*

MENOPAUSE:

Lachesis for hot flashes and fainting; Worse with tight clothing.
Lilium Tig for intensity, depression, irritability and prolapse.
Pulsatilla when clingy, complaining, weepy and sad; Worse with heat.
Sepia when overwhelmedand irritable; Prefers solitude; Hot flashes.
Consider: *Sulphur; Natrum Mur; Phosphorus; Sabina; Kreosotum.*

MENSES:

Absent: Aurum; Ferrum; Graphites; Kali Carb; Lycopodium; Puls.
Clotted: Belladonna; Calcarea; China; Lachesis; Sabina; Puls.
Cramps: Chamomilla; Cocculus; Colocynthis; Mag Phos; Sepia.
Frequent: Arsenicum; Belladonna; Cyclamen; Ferrum; Phos.
Irregular: Argent Nit; Nux Moschata; Puls; Sepia; Senecio.
Late: Causticum; Cuprum; Lachesis; Natrum Mur; Sarsparilla.
Painful: Cimicifuga; Mag Phos; Millefolium; Cactus; Puls; Sabina; Sulphur; Caulophyllum; Cyclamen; Chamomilla.
Profuse: Arsenicum; Ferrum Phos; Phos; Calcarea Phos; Sabina; Senecio; Millefolium; Natrum Mur; Ferrum; Cyclamen.
Suppressed: Belladonna; Cyclamen; Lachesis; Senecio; Sepia.

PELVIC INFLAMMATORY DISEASE:

Arsenicum for burning, offensive discharge with anxiety.

Lac Caninum for ovarian pains and vaginal gas; Fear of snakes.

Lachesis for left-sided pains and cysts; Worse with tight clothing.

Sabina for severe PMS, intense pains, gushing flow; Leukorrhea.

Consider: *Apis; Belladonna; Cantharis; Puls; Chamomilla; Sepia.*

VAGINITIS:

Medorrhinum for high sex drive and chronic infection; Herpes.

Pulsatilla when needy and capricious; Does not tolerate pain.

Thuja for green discharges, herpes, polyps and cysts.

Kreosotum for strong itch with burning discharge and odor.

Consider: *Arsenicum; Graphites; Mercurious; Sepia; Sulphur.*

The remedies and disharmonies described in this section reflect only a portion of the totality. Labels such as "Sports Injuries" are limiting and do not express the individual picture required to choose a remedy. *It is best not to use these limited remedy pictures and labels alone.* Take a complete case and use this section as a guideline.

These short remedy descriptions provide a starting point for determining the most effective remedy. Also, the remedies described under each heading are the primary ones used for these disharmonies, but not all remedies are included.

There are many acute problems which are not discussed in this chapter. Those described are the most often mentioned when requiring first aid or treatment.

Acute illnesses are similar to a leaky faucet, in that they are rarely serious, they just seem so. It may take a new fitting or pipe, but recovery is quick and most times, permanent. Remedies can provide the same relief.

A discussion on chronic problems is in the next chapter, These illnesses frequently require assistance from a health care provider, as symptoms and etiology are complex and often interrelated. Poor choice of a remedy can cause greater harm as it may cover symptoms which need further evaluation.

Chapter Eight

Chronic Illness: The Long Term

The following presentation is for the purpose of education. It is to be used as a guide in further understanding the difficulty which arises with long-term illnesses.

Defining chronic illness as a disharmony in the body that lasts for longer than ten days is easy. Understanding the cause is far more difficult. There is much more to the term "chronic" than just duration.

In illness of this nature, labels are used to define problems, such as asthma or insomnia. This is not the entire picture, as labels only tend to reflect a manifestation of deeper disharmonies, and usually relate to underlying causes. Homeopathy looks more to the cause of the illness rather than the label, as treating the cause will almost always eliminate the resulting problem.

Often, though, the cause is not clear. Concise casetaking can help you determine underlying disharmonies by understanding the individual and his or her history. A chronic case can have several layers of manifestation, such as grief on the emotional level, an accident on the physiological level and inability to concentrate on the mental level.

As mentioned earlier, all layers interrelate and an inability to concentrate may stem from a head injury in an auto accident. Grief may go much deeper and have endured for a longer time. Symptoms which are most dominant in the moment are the ones addressed at the outset. These are the most limiting symptoms and are unique to each person.

There are times when the selected remedy brings about balance even for the deepest and most chronic disharmony because it fits the person, rather than just their illness. In every case, the essence and the totality is important, not just labels or pathology. Remedy selection encompasses all facets.

There are also times when a remedy seems to fit the person, their disharmony, and even their strongest presenting symptoms yet still has little effect. Why? Several reasons usually factor into the equation, the most obvious of which is an inaccurate remedy selection, requiring further evaluation. Another possibility centers on obstacles to cure when someone is reluctant to change their habits, such as eliminating coffee or learning to adapt to stress. A third consideration concerns recent layers or traumas which aren't being fully addressed in the remedy selection. This may effectively block the remedy from reaching its potential.

A well-chosen remedy that relates to the totality of the individual works regardless of potency or energy blocks and even despite various obstacles, so the first reason is frequently the culprit. It takes several years to feel comfortable with remedy selections and as is so often the case, information acquired from poorly chosen remedies helps with future casetaking.

A permanent cure for chronic illnesses can be difficult, especially when it has lasted for a long time. For instance, skin disharmonies that have caused problems for years can take over a year or more to clear while the same is true for most long-term illness. It is important to disregard standard philosophies for immediate healing and endeavor to persevere with whatever time is required for recovery.

As described previously, there is a responsibility to explain that energy and the vital force heal in their own time and in their own unique manner. Homeopathy can be a subtle healing force that brings balance to the body. If the illness did not occur overnight, then cure or balance will not come from taking the first dose of the remedy. This is not magic or a magic pill, but rather, a means of healing and elimination which touch the deepest levels of the entire human system.

Each step is carefully monitored, from the initial casetaking process to evaluation and analysis. These are followed by effective case management and frequent reevaluation. With each step there is improvement, change and ongoing recovery. The same remedy may be used throughout the entire process, changing and increasing potency as needed, or a new remedy picture may present itself requiring a different selection.

The idea is to be open to presenting and current symptoms, those which stand out from the others. Basically, it is more of a reflection of what remedy the body is asking for at that specific time. It may not come from words alone, it might be certain mannerisms, or a voice inflection, or appearance, or even a subtle attitude that can provide a clue to a specific remedy.

It is important to fully observe all aspects of a case while making clear, accurate notes. The use of quotation marks when unique statements are made helps during the analysis process. This creates a written transcript of the initial interview and is useful for follow-up visits and reevaluation. Continued evaluations allow the chronic illness to become manageable and less threatening.

There are thousands of chronic problems, some made up of combinations of disharmonies, creating larger pictures of discomfort and disease. The following are a few of the labels used to describe these diseases. Use the selections as a starting point rather than an ultimate selection for recovery.

ASTHMA:

Arsenicum when anxious, obsessive, chilled, restless, and worried; burning sensations; worse between 11 p.m. and 1 a.m.; better with heat.

Kali Carbonicum for a hypersensitive, rigid type with a strong moral sense; worse between 2 and 5 a.m.; better when bending forward.

Medorrhinum for childhood asthma; hurried, restless; extremists; eczema; warm; clears throat a lot; worse a.m., better nighttime.

Sulphur has skin problems, more mental than emotional, indolent and messy; warm-blooded; worse when standing or too warm in bed.

Consider: *Tuberculinum; Thuja; Phosphorus; Natrum Sulf; Silica.*

BACKACHE:

Bryonia for those times that pain is intensified with any motion; stiffness; is irritable; prefers to be alone; worse in cold and better with heat.

Causticum has slow paralysis, cervical tension, hard tendons and warts; an intense/idealistic personality; compulsive; holds onto old grief.

Ranunculus Bulbosus is worse when cold, damp or walking; sore muscles; stiffness and stabbing pains; depressed about condition.

Rhus Tox has restlessness, stiffness and sciatica; better continued motion and stretching; pain is better with heat, hot bath and pressure.

Consider: *Ruta; Nux Vomica; Sulphur; Sepia; Silica; Calcarea; Ledum.*

CANCER:

Breast: Asterias; Conium; Graphites; Hydrastis; Phytolaca; Silica.

Bones: Calcarea Fluor; Conium; Hecla lava; Phosphorus; Symphytum.

Colon: Alumina; Arsenicum; Hydrastis; Kali Carb; Nitric Acid; Sepia.

Hodgkin's: Arsenicum; Calcarea Flour; Carcinosin; Phytolaca; Thuja.

Leukemia: Arsenicum; Calcarea; China; Natrum Ars; Natrum Sulf.

Lung: Arsenicum; Carcinosin; Conium; Phosphorus; Sulphur; Thuja.

Ovarian: Conium; Graphites; Kreosotum; Lachesis; Medorrhinum.

Pancreatic: Calcarea Ars; Conium; Hydrastis; Phosphorus; Spongia.

Prostate: Carcinosin; Conium; Iodum; Selenium; Silica; Sulphur.

Skin: Arsenicum; Conium; Hydrastis; Kreosotum; Lycopodium; Silica.

CHRONIC FATIGUE:

Ammonium Carb has brain fag, exhaustion and poor endurance; worse in cold weather; often cardiac symptoms coincide.

Carcinosin is often worse since having mononucleosis, with a history of family cancer; passionate; perfectionist; worried; worse between 1 and 6 p.m.

Phosphoric Acid when emotionally exhausted; grief, shock and unhappy love; mild person; indifferent and lazy.

Picric Acid is averse to thinking or talking; worse exertion; dull mind, weak memory; strong sexual desire; worse with heat; better with cold.

Consider: *Arsenicum; China; Gelsemium; Ferrum; Scutellaria; Silica.*

HERPES ZOSTER:

Arsenicum is anxious about their health, has small, white, scaly flaking and burning sensations; better in summer; skin is better with heat.

Iris has right-sided Zoster with gastric problems; eruptions come in patches and on elbows and knees; thin, delicate, nervous, sweet type.

Mezereum has cracks that ooze and crust over; burning, shooting pains; neuralgic pains remain after shingles disappear; anxious.

Rhus Tox for eruptions that burn and itch; related joint problems; restless; sad; worse when cold; better in hot water; better when stretching.
Consider: *Alnus; Graphites; Petroleum; Natrum Mur; Sulphur; Sepia.*

OBESITY:

Calcarea has slow metabolism, is overly responsible, fearful and anxious; flabby; late develop.m.ent as child; worse exertion; chilly.

Capsicum is lazy, chilly, hypersensitive, rigid, clumsy; burning pains; gets bored and homesick easily; worse with change or with heat.

Ferrum has capricious moods, sensitivity to noise and likes to be alone; flushed face; chilly; restless; abusive; better with gentle motion.

Graphites is full of doubts, unable to make decisions, has low self-esteem and is fastidious; anxious; chilly; skin problems; excitable.
Consider: *Pulsatilla; Phytolacca; Fucus; Ammonium Mur; Kali Carb.*

ORGANS/GLANDS:

Adrenals: Arsenicum; Calcarea Ars; Ammonium Brom; Sepia; Adren.

Bladder: Apis; Cantheris; Lycopodium; Sarsparilla; Berberis; Equis.

Brain: Alumina; Belladonna; Conium; Phosphorus; Helleborus; Nux V.

Gallbladder: Berberis; China; Cardus M; Natrum Sulf; Veratrum A.

Heart: Aurum; Crataegus; Lachesis; Phosphorus; Naja; Cactus; Lith.

Kidney: Berberis; Cantheris; Equistium; Lycopodium; Natrum M; Phos.

Liver: Arsenicum; Cardus M; Chelidonium; Nux Vomica; Cornus; Phos.

Lungs: Blatta; Lobelia; Kali Carb; Arsenicum; Sambucus; Thuja; Sulf.

Pancreas: Conium; Iris; Mercurius; Phosphorus; Spongia; Iodum.

Spleen: Arsenicum; Asafoetida; Ceanothus; China; Sulfuric Acid; Ign.

Thyroid: Bromium; Calcarea; Iodum; Natrum Mur; Sepia; Spongia.

PSYCHOLOGICAL:

Abandonment: Argent N; Aurum; Natrum Carb; Pulsatilla; Psorinum.

Abusive: Anacardium; Aurum; Chamomilla; Hepar; Lachesis; Nux V.

Anger: Anacardium; Bryonia; Cina; Ignacia; Lycopodium; Nitric Acid; Sepia; Staphysagria; Sulphur; Chamomilla; Natrum Mur; Nux Vomica.

Anxiety: Aconite; Argent N; Arsenicum; Aurum; Belladonna; Bryonia; Calcarea; Camphor; Carcinosin; Causticum; China; Natrum Carb; Phos; Psorinum; Pulsatilla; Rhus Tox; Veratrum A; Sulphur; Nitric Acid.

Confidence (low): Anacardium; Aurum; Baryta Carb; Calcarea F; Carcinosin; Kali Phos; Lycopodium; Natrum Mur; Psorinum; Silica; Staphysagria; Pulsatilla; Thuja; Nux Vomica; China; Lac Caninum.

Critical: Arsenicum; Graphites; Sulphur; Veratrum A; Chamomilla; Bromium; Lachesis; Lycopodium; Mercurius; Nux Vomica; Sepia; Phos.

Depression: Aconite; Arsenicum; Aurum; Calcarea; Carcinosin; Carcinosin; Causticum; China; Ferrum; Graphites; Iodum; Ignacia; Lachesis; Natrum Mur, Carb and Sulf; Nitric Acid; Platina; Rhus Tox; Psorinum; Pulsatilla; Sepia; Sulphur; Thuja; Veratrum A; Zincum.

Domineering: Anacardium; Lycopodium; China; Lachesis; Mercurius; Platina; Sulphur; Cuprum; Camphor; Veratrum A; Arsenicum Album.

Fastidious: Arsenicum; Anacardium; Carcinosin; Graphites; Natrum Mur and Sulf; Lycopodium; Nux Vomica; Pulsatilla; Silica.

Fear: Aconite; Argentum N; Arsenicum; Aurum; Calcarea; Carcinosin; Graphites; Ignacia; Kali A; Lycopodium; Natrum Carb; Phosphorus; Platina; Psorinum; Sepia; Stramonium; Zincum Phos.

Grief: Aurum; Carcinosin; Causticum; Cocculus; Ignacia; Lachesis; Natrum Mur; Nux Vomica; Phosphoric Acid; Phosphorus; Staphysagria.

Guilt: Aluminum; Arsenicum; Aurum; Carcinosin; Chelidonium; Digitalis; Natrum Mur; Psorinum; Staphysagria; Sulphur; Causticum.

Indifference: Aluminum; Anacardium; Apis; Calcarea; China; Lilium Tig; Gelsemium; Natrum Carb, Mur and Phos; Nux Vomica; Phosphorus;Phosphoric Acid; Platina; Pulsatilla; Sepia; Staphysagria; Zincum.

Irritability: Antimonium Crudum; Arsenicum; Belladonna; Bryonia; Calcarea; Chamomilla; Graphites; Hepar; Lilium Tig; Lycopodium; Nux Vomica; Natrum Carb and Mur; Nitric Acid; Phosphoric Acid; Phos; Petrolium; Platina; Rhus Tox; Pulsatilla; Sepia; Silica; Staphysagria.

Jealousy: Apis; Causticum; Hyoscyamus; Kali Carb; Lachesis; Nux Vomica; Lycopodium; Medorrhinum; Platina; Pulsatilla; Stramonium.

Laziness: Carbo Sulf; Chelidonium; China; Graphites; Lachesis; Nux Vomica; Lycopodium; Natrum Mur; Nitric Acid; Phosphorus; Picric Acid; Pulsatilla; Sulphur; Tuberculinum; Zincum Phos.

Memory (Poor): Baryta C; Carbo Sulf; Cocculus; Colchicum; Platina; Lycopodium; Mercurius; Petrolium; Phosphoric Acid; Phosphorous.

Obsessive: Anacardium; Argentum N; Arsenicum; Calcarea; Nux Vomica; Carcinosin; Hyoscyamos; Medorrhinum; Natrum Mur and Sulf; Platina; Pulsatilla; Silica; Staphysagria; Veratrum A.

Obstinate: Aluminum; Anacardium; Argentricum N; Bryonia; Cina; Calcarea; Chamomilla; Nux Vomica; Tarantula; Tuberculinum; Thuja.

Passive: Arsenicum; Baryta Carb; Ignacia; Lycopodium; Natrum M; Phosphorus; Pulsatilla; Silica; Staphysagria; Aurum.

Pessimistic: Arsenicum; Aurum; Nitric Acid; Nux V; Psorinum.

Quarrelsome: Aurum; Chamomilla; Cina; Hyoscyamos; Nux Vomica; Petroleum; Sepia; Silica; Sulphur; Tarantula; Thuja; Natrum Mur.

Rage: Agaricus; Anacardium; Belladonna; Cantharis; Hyoscyamos; Lac Caninum; Lachesis; Lycopodium; Moschus; Nux V; Stramonium.

Restless: Aconite; Anacardium; Argentum N; Arsenicum; Baptisia; Calcarea P; Camphora; Carcinosin; Cimicifuga; Colocynthis; Cuprum; Ferrum; Helleborus; Lycopodium; Medorrhinum; Mercurius; Rhus Tox; Sepia; Silica; Staphysagria; Stramonium; Sulphur; Tarantula.

Sensitive (Hyper): Causticum; Natrum Carb, Mur and Phos; Lilium Tig; Silica; Staphysagria; Asarum; Coffea; Aurum; Chamomilla; Phosphorus.

Suicidal: Aurum; Aurum Met; Natrum Sulf; Psorinum; China; Natrum Mur; Lachesis; Stramonium; Zincum; Nux V; Arsenicum; Anacardium.

Suspicious: Aconite; Anacardium; Arsenicum; Baryta Carb; Bryonia; Causticum; Lachesis; Lycopodium; Pulsatilla; Rhus Tox; Stramonium.

Sympathetic: Calcarea P; Carcinosin; Causticum; Cocculus; Ignacia; Natrum Carb and Mur; Nitric Acid; Nux V; Phosphorus; Pulsatilla.

Talk (Loquacity): Aurum; Cocculus; Hyoscyamos; Lachesis; Moschus; Stramonium; Natrum Carb; Phosphorus; Veratrum A.

Timid: Baryta Carb; Bryonia; Calcarea; Gelsemium; Kali C; Natrum Carb; Lycopodium; Petroleum; Phosphorus; Silica;

Pulsatilla; Sepia; Staphysagria; Sulphur; Tuberculinum; Arsenicum; Aurum; Causticum.

Violent: Anacardium; Aurum; Belladonna; Cicuta;
Hyoscyamos; Nux Vomica; Lachesis; Natrum M; Petroleum;
Stramonium; Tuberculinum.

Weary: Arsenicum; Aurum; Carcinosin; China; Kali P; Natrum
Mur and Sulph; Mercurious; Nitric Acid; Nux V; Phosphoric
Acid; Phosphorus.

Worry: Arsenicum; Calcarea; Causticum; China; Ignacia;
Lycopodium; Natrum Carb and Mur; Phosphoric Acid;
Pulsatilla; Staphysagria.

SLEEP (INSOMNIA):

Chamomilla is restless in early morning; irritable and
needs to walk.

Coffea has an active mind and is worse from surprising
news.

Nux Vomica is worse after mental strain or overindulgence.

Rhus Tox needs to constantly shift in bed; nothing is
comfortable.

Consider: *Arsenicum; Argentum N; Bryonia; Kali C; Lachesis; Silica.*

STRESS:

Argentum Nit has fear and apprehension before any event;
panics easily.

Gelsemium is mentally paralyzed from stage fright or
exams.

Passaflora provides a quieting effect on the nervous
system.

Valeriana can calm restlessness; oversensitive and moody.

Consider: *Aconite; Chamomilla; Ignacia; Natrum M; Nux
V; Pulsatilla.*

As previously stated, and which cannot be overempha-
sized, the above descriptions and remedies are only a minor
aspect of casetaking. Do not use short cuts or pathology

alone, take the case and understand the person, not just their symptoms.

There is a phrase in homeopathy which states "the person, not the cure". This means the person, in his or her totality, will reflect the correct and necessary remedy at that moment. Therefore, the cure is secondary to the individual response. A cure will come in its time, yet balance and the general sense of well-being that arises before the actual cure is the basis of homeopathy.

Chronic imbalance is curable with effort, patience, intention and education. By allowing enough time in the beginning, each person will begin to trust the process necessary for recovery and healing. During this time trust develops between the person and the homeopath. This relationship requires mutual respect and compassion, yet it also requires time and effort from both parties. Follow-up consultations and evaluations establish a deeper understanding of pathology, personality and etiology.

Often, in our society, individuals are accustomed to and demand immediate results. In homeopathy, the healing is often more subtle, but does not suppress or mask symptoms. For this reason, as mentioned above, the need to provide information about duration of remedies, aggravations, antidoting and what can be expected after taking the remedy is important and necessary.

Without using this procedure, an individual will not understand why old symptoms have returned, or why their symptoms have become worse, or why there has been no change of any kind, or even why they may need to have a follow-up evaluation.

Chronic problems may well be inherited tendencies, which require special evaluation and procedures. In any case, use caution in prescribing remedies, especially in high potencies. And under no circumstance should a remedy be prescribed based on a single symptom like asthma, as a proving may result and further harm could arise. A proving of this kind can create unrelated symptoms which only confound the results.

Excellent results can be obtained by following the procedures outlined in the previous chapters. We do not take a car apart without having some knowledge of how to put it back together. In homeopathy, we do not give a remedy without knowing the probable effect it will have on the entire human system as confirmed by past provings.

Case management follows as a means of reviewing a case after the first dose and after the first effect. As with each of the preceding parts, certain procedures help in the follow-up evaluation and analysis, especially when the remedy has not been as effective as needed.

Chapter Nine

Case Management: The Follow-up

The initial casetaking and remedy selection are the first steps necessary to determine which follow-up approach to take. This includes changing the potency, repeating the same remedy at the same potency or possibly selecting a new remedy. But what is to be done after the second consultation if the first well-chosen remedy has not been effective.

This step can be very important, as the second remedy should be carefully selected and given *only* when no change has occurred since the first dose. Reinterrogation and reevaluation of symptoms, reactions, results, new or old symptoms, improvement or deterioration are invaluable at this point. The purpose is to judge the impact of the remedy or even lack of impact and how best to proceed. Also, this review helps to discover whether or not the person has accidentally, or even intentionally, antidoted the remedy.

Why would someone intentionally antidote their remedy? Perhaps there was an intense aggravation from a too high of a potency. Or, on further thought, they realized that they were not quite ready to go through any aggravation as their existing patterns/symptoms were still acceptable. Possibly they were unable to give up coffee, marijuana, alcohol, street drugs or aromatherapy.

It is difficult to always know how an individual will react to a remedy as each person releases old symptoms in their own unique way. By explaining possible reactions at the outset, the person becomes aware of the outcome and has less of a desire to antidote. Remember when you first learned how to ride a bike and your teacher helped hold the bike upright, allowing you to pedal and go fast, while telling you to that you were safe. There was some fear, but the assistance and explanation helped reduce the unknown factors, much like an explanation before taking a remedy.

Also, keeping to the lower potencies until experience and knowledge has increased will help in eliminating intense aggravations.

The information from the asthma case can help to further clarify case management processes as well as the second consultation. In reviewing a case after taking the remedy, an individual's symptom picture becomes clearer in conjunction with the remedy response.

In the follow-up consultation, the first question asked refers to any changes noticed after taking the remedy. Request that the response be as explicit and complete as possible. The term *change* is important, as it encompasses both *improvement and aggravation*. As noted previously, leading questions about changes or symptoms are not valuable during this procedure, as they prevent spontaneous thoughts and feelings. Perceptions about changes and symptoms are often very insightful and can provide a glimpse into causes.

Returning to the previously described asthma case, the following is his answer to the question about changes after taking the remedy. He noticed some initial difficulty in his breathing, especially at night around 4 a.m. However, his breathing improved after three days and has stabilized since. He also talked about the following symptoms:

1. He seems to be able to get a deeper breath than before.
2. He feels a bit less angry while not being triggered as easily.
3. His desire for sweets has diminished somewhat, although the effort is more conscious on his part.
4. He still is overly critical and worries about money.
5. He didn't think there were any other changes.

Considering that 40 days have elapsed since the first visit, this shows an awareness of several changes. Often, a follow-up review reflects that not much has happened since taking the remedy and it is not until specific questions are asked from the initial interview material that they realize specific

Case Management: The Follow-up

changes have occurred. That's why good initial note-taking is important, otherwise reevaluation based on memory alone is almost impossible.

The second question to ask is whether or not there have been any new symptoms that have arisen since taking the remedy. The purpose is to find out if a proving has taken place and if so, to what degree. This is obviously avoided by the careful selection of the remedy based on presenting symptoms. Aggravations may arise, but rarely a proving, when a close remedy is chosen.

Next, question the person about any old symptoms returning from previous illnesses or traumas. From this response, a determination can be made as to the depth of the remedy reaction. The term *old* means symptoms that existed in childhood or anytime before their current symptoms arose. When asked this question, the person with asthma reflected and felt that there were no old symptoms.

This suggests either the remedy is only going to be effective on the more current symptom picture or the potency was not high enough to resonate with older ones. Be careful with asthma or life-threatening situations, or even debilitating diseases. Potencies which are too high can aggravate or overstimulate the disharmony. *If in doubt, stay with the lower potencies, such as a 12c, and repeat as necessary.*

As noted from the initial question in the follow-up, he stated that there were some minor aggravations after taking the first dose, but these quickly dissipated, so the potency was not too high. Anything 30c or lower is usually fine in cases of this nature.

Reviewing the initial symptom picture, as described at the first consultation, is the next step in understanding the remedy reaction. The key elements of the first casetaking are specifically addressed here, along with any unique symptoms used in choosing the first remedy. It is not necessary at this point to review symptoms mentioned in the follow-up consultation, unless they are new or previously unexpressed.

Frequently, someone describes old symptoms remembered after the first visit. These are often quite helpful. Also, if there is a question or lack of clarity regarding any changes described, then have the person explain their symptoms or feelings in more detail.

The asthma case initially had 22 rubrics. These were reduced to 10 symptoms, and from these 10 rubrics, the remedy was selected. In reviewing the stronger and more limiting symptoms from the first visit, he says that he is not quite as chilly, although the weather has been warmer so he probably would not notice the cold as much. This is a common response, where an individual justifies improvement or change with another related occurrence. Measure the change cautiously, but do not disregard it.

When asked about his controlling tendencies, he says that he has not noticed any difference, which is the same response he gives for his aggravation from the wind. Also, no old symptoms relating to his suppressed venereal disease have returned.

Do not forget about any observations made at the first interview, especially something like restlessness. Does the person seem more calm, less fidgety and active? Keep notes on their behavior, for even if no change is noticed on this visit, perhaps a future one may reflect a shift.

After going over all the important symptoms previously mentioned, ask about sleep patterns, dreams, digestion, food desires, relationships, motivation and anything else that may seem different in their lives. This information, in conjunction with the symptom material, creates a basis for reevaluation and analysis.

As shown above, there were some definite changes described in the asthma case follow-up. Improvement was reflected on both the physical and emotional levels which shows that the remedy did have some effect, but it may have only been palliative. Is the remedy repeated at a higher dose, the same dose, or is it necessary to just wait?

Case Management: The Follow-up

The answer depends on the potency given and when improvement began to relapse. For this individual, 40 days have elapsed since taking the remedy and it continues to hold for both the emotional anger and the pathology of asthma. In addition, vital heat and lack of chilliness may have changed while there is less craving for sweets. So no repetition is needed, nor should one be given, even with a low potency like a 30c dilution. Let the remedy run its course, for however long it does. To paraphrase an old adage, if it's still working don't try to fix it. This applies to repetition of remedies as well.

When, and if, the symptoms do return, regardless of time, give the same potency again. If a remedy is working and has worked for an extended period, do not change it or go to a higher potency. Give it time to reach its potential and do all it possibly can before moving on to another remedy or potency.

According to Kent, the second remedy is the one given after the first has acted. In other words, if four remedies have been taken by the person and none have been effective, while the fifth one given has acted, then the fifth remedy is actually the first, because it acted.

Many homeopaths contend that unless an aggravation arises from the first acting remedy, then it is an incorrect choice. Duration of these aggravations would be unimportant, just as long as there was a release of old symptoms.

As there are always exceptions to any given maxim, be aware that an aggravation does not arise in every instance. Original symptoms can reappear without aggravation and be of short duration. This return of symptoms may bring to mind similar occurrences from one's past, which is a good sign of release. Intense or severe aggravations may be uniquely limited, depending on the individual and past symptoms. It is the general well-being of the person, and observations of those changes, which provides the basis for analysis and evaluation.

Hahnemann discusses this phenomena in the Oragnon when he reflects on his approach to healing: "The highest ideal of homeopathic therapy is to restore health rapidly, gently and permanently." Underlying this concept is the ideal of assisting the patient with recovery in the safest manner without causing aggravation or overstimulation.

Case management is often more difficult than the choice of the first remedy, as it requires patience and perseverance. The key words are: *watch and wait*. If a remedy is repeated too quickly or a new one chosen before the first remedy has been exhausted, then the picture may become muddled. Guiding symptoms to the next remedy are created only upon completion of the first, and without guiding symptoms, clarity and choice are often prevented.

In the final analysis, the effect of the first remedy is always given the greatest weight. Insignificant changes may suggest something more superficial and are not as strongly considered.

For instance, the individual with asthma had a better ability to breathe with less anger. These represent two strong symptoms. If they had not improved or changed in any way, then a reevaluation would consider a different remedy for those specific symptoms. Effective changes require a "wait and see" approach before repeating or revising, but with no important changes occurring after taking a remedy, reconsider the first selection.

Without clear presenting symptoms, there is nothing upon which to choose a remedy. And without waiting for clarity to surface, the remedy picture remains unclear and ineffective.

Remember, the return of old symptoms is an excellent indicator of a well-chosen remedy, but rarely is the core or essence of a case reached with just a single remedy.

When the first acting remedy has ceased its action entirely and has been exhausted by several repetitions, then guiding symptoms provide a clear direction to the next remedy. If someone is trying to find their way by the stars and it's a clear night, the journey is easy. If there are clouds obscuring the stars, the journey becomes quite difficult and arduous. With strong symptoms and clear direction, the remedy becomes obvious.

Some cases are obviously more difficult than others and they require different skills. Layer upon layer of disharmony tends to create unusual symptom pictures, some of which need to be peeled off one at a time. Each case is evaluated on its own merit and range of discomfort. Symptoms creating severe pain, either emotional or physical, are addressed first, so as to establish a return to joy and health.

Evaluating difficult cases follows in the next chapter, with the caution that an effective analysis is important before selecting a remedy.

Chapter Ten

Difficult Cases: An Evaluation

In the early stages of studying homeopathy, there is a new ideal for both health and healing. These concepts, philosophies and approaches are quite formative and appealing to many individuals. Experience, study, casetaking and time help alleviate the early sense of confusion and doubt. Feeling overwhelmed is a part of the process in learning any new complex subject.

In the beginning, working with acute cases helps to establish an understanding of the principles and precepts of homeopathic material, while achieving a satisfactory number of successful cases. Afterwards, complex cases can help you develop homeopathic skills and understanding on deeper levels.

Much like a mystery novel, difficult cases provide all the aspects one could hope for in discovering who or what did it. There are intrigues, clues, histories, questions, double-meanings, suspects, causes and conclusions. The goal is to solve the mystery while locating the most similar remedy, given the guiding symptoms in the moment.

Multilayers or traumas are the primary components of most difficult cases, but predispositions and inherited tendencies play a large role in untangling the intrigue.

First, it is valuable to discover what it is about this particular case that makes it difficult or unusual. It helps to organize each symptom according to patterns and chronological stages.

The following describes a 30-year-old woman with various levels of disharmony, occurring at different times in her life. Each level of her case can be evaluated and listed in order of appearing symptoms. The greater the disharmony, the more important the symptom becomes in finding the closest remedy. In other words, what is presently the most limiting aspect of her life? Her symptoms include:

1. Family history of disease, cancer (predisposition).
2. A suppression in childhood (use of steroids for eczema).
3. A trauma (sexual abuse).
4. A major loss and sustained grief (Mother dies at age 9).
5. The first menses was traumatic and has been worse since.
6. Has been worse since a trip to India (contracted worms).
7. Everything has intensified since the birth of her first child.

A graph follows, but first give each trauma or pathology its own time line, from birth to the present time, such as: number two line from age 2 through age 4; number three from age 6 to age 10; number 4 from age nine to the present; number 5 from age 13 through the present; number 6 from age 19 through the present; number 7 from age 24 to the present. It would look something like this:

age 2-4 (eczema)

age 6-10 (sexual abuse)

age 9-30 (mother's death, continued grief and loss)

age 13-30 (traumatic and continuing menses problems)

age 19-30 (worms or parasites)

age 24-30 (birth of a child)

prebirth to present (possible predisposition to cancer)

Use time line number one, predisposition to cancer, only if there are current symptoms related to the inherited tendency. For instance, ovarian cysts, warts, moles or growths of any sort. In this case, such symptoms do exist since birth and is the last line drawn above. Note that this is the line which covers the entire lifetime.

It helps to create this time line in the casetaking process, but for now, get a piece of paper and draw a line for each period, dating it from beginning to end. The longest lines reflect time periods that are strongly considered in the final evaluation. These lines indicate disharmony which has endured despite additional traumas and injuries. These are the deeper aspects and require attention and inclusion in the remedy choice.

The initial analysis is important at this point, as the difficulty arises from the degree and severity of existing symptoms. When many symptoms intertwine and interact as these do, determining which are the causative ones becomes important.

There are two long time lines to consider, the first, or the predisposition to cancer and the long-term grief from the loss of her mother. Sexual abuse and menstrual disharmony since the first menses will also be included, depending on how they continue to impact her current life.

To summarize, the patient is a 30-year-old woman with a history of cancer and specific predispostions. She has suppressed eczema, sexual abuse at age 6, loss of her mother at age 9, has never felt the same since her first menses, has been worse since travel to India and even worse since the birth of her first child.

What symptoms should be considered as important and necessary? Her current chief complaint or the most limiting aspect in her life is the first place to look. In this example, only the key symptoms are provided but let us assume her chief complaint is chronic fatigue. By evaluating this symptom along with her other presenting symptoms, we begin to get a picture of the possible cause.

She has had chronic fatigue since her trip to India but it has become worse since the birth of her child. Further questioning will assist in the analysis here, but a general assumption would probably indicate that the fatigue began much earlier, perhaps even from the time of her mother's death. It may not have been as severe as it currently is, but on further questioning, she states that she was always tired to some degree or another from the age of six.

What happened when she was six? She was molested by an uncle who came over frequently to help her sick mother. It is here that the underlying cause may exist, along with her predisposition to cancer and the suppressed eczema. All her symptoms appear to be interrelated, some to a greater degree than others, but each is a factor in the final analysis.

Discovering the cause in each case is very helpful, but not always possible. The time line approach can assist in the event that cause is not clear. It also provides the thread that runs throughout the entire lifetime, such as the her cancer symptoms.

What then is to be used in the selection of a remedy? Chronic fatigue is the presenting symptom picture and will be included. It is important to always address the chief complaint, as that is the primary reason for the consultation. The underlying cause was the sexual abuse, or at the very least, it was from this point that the loss of energy became a factor. This is also included in the final mix. Being as the cancer symptoms have existed since birth, it would be safe to consider those as well.

With these three symptoms, sexual abuse, chronic fatigue and a cancer predisposition, there is a good picture of the presenting complaint and its cause. From this alone, several remedies come to mind (Carcinosin, Natrum Muriaticum, Sepia), but to get a complete representation, mental aspects and the totality must be noted. The purpose here was to assist in dissecting a difficult case rather than analyze or prescribe a remedy.

Without taking a full case, it would be a disservice to choose a remedy based on a limited symptom picture. Poor casetaking and analysis only lead to minor relief of symptoms, along with possible ill effects and discord. In that regard, most individuals will ultimately become disillusioned with homeopathy and its potential.

Some additional aspects need to be discussed about difficult cases, including layers, miasms, obstacles and recovery.

Layers of trauma may require specific treatment procedures for each specific layer. For instance, consider that the above abuse case did not respond to the first remedy, despite time and effort to assess the situation as a whole. Several factors would be considered:

1. The remedy was not the correct one and reevaluation is necessary.
2. The most recent layer is "blocking" access to the cause.
3. An undefined layer is limiting recovery.
4. The remedy was antidoted or the potency was too low.
5. The underlying predisposition needs to be "cleared."

Being as homeopathy is not an exact science, there are times when a well-chosen remedy has no impact, simply as a result of one of the above situations. Keep that remedy selection in mind, but decide on the next best approach, such as the most recent layer first and work backwards. For instance, the woman described above has been worse since the birth of her child, but the fatigue had gotten worse after the trip to India and before the birth of the child.

Begin with the India trip and consider the whole in light of that aspect. Track the progress. Guiding symptoms should arise to provide a direction for each succeeding remedy. If there is no improvement after several remedies, consider working with the miasm. These are the inherited predispositions related to specific symptom pictures. The next chapter will address miasms in further detail.

The two final components for difficult cases—obstacles to a cure and the recovery process—can be understood by delving further into family history, daily tendencies, habits, relationships, career, stress and expression of emotions.

Complete review of obstacles to cure is addressed in a later chapter.

Recovery in difficult cases deals primarily with the duration of the healing process. It takes time for the person's system to find its own level of balance. Recovery may be slow or subtle. If decades have created the disharmony, healing will also take time, perhaps even several years. But, there is continued improvement over that period and the need for honesty about this possible time frame and healing process allows each individual to develop trust and patience.

Difficult cases and their intertwining mysteries can be the most rewarding work a homeopath does, especially when a person rediscovers health and well-being. Rarely is it time alone that assists in recovering this balance, but more, it is about the joy and happiness a person is able to rediscover.

Chapter Eleven

Miasms: An Inherited Tendency

D octor Hahnemann developed his theory on miasms to explain various contagious diseases, especially chronic ones. Included in his ideas for possible contaminants and causes were syphilis, scabies, gonorrhea, tuberculosis and fevers such as typhoid and cholera.

His hypothesis predated any known material on bacteria and parasites, despite the fact there were no microscopes in his day. Many have claimed that Hahnemann is the Father of Bacteriology, and rightly so. According to Hahnemann, the cause of chronic disease was micro-organisms.

The word "miasma" is derived from the Greek, meaning stain or pollution. It has evolved to mean predisposition to chronic disease, whether inherited or developed early on in life. This disease state can be transmitted from generation to generation through genetics and suppressions.

If a chronic disease has been suppressed in any manner, it is retained in the organism, creating a greater susceptibility in succeeding generations. With each passing generation, susceptibility grows stronger and the inherent weakness, greater. Cancer would appear to be the current manifestation of this phenomenon, what with its increased incidence and proliferation in society.

An inherited immune system that is unable to combat disease, germs or viruses will ultimately succumb to those disharmonies. Our body is constantly in a struggle with bacteria and germs, a minute by minute mini-war, which requires a fortified immune system. Working with miasms and inherent predispositions, homeopathy can release these weaknesses and strengthen the immune system.

During his lifetime, Hahnemann worked with three distinct miasms which he called psoric, sycotic and syphilitic. The tubercular miasm was later added by homeopaths, allegedly being a combination of psoric and syphilitic tendencies. In fact, it is not really a combination at all, as tuberculosis preceded syphilis on the European Continent. Syphilis was established on the Continent only after Columbus' travels to the New World. Recently a cancer miasm has been discussed and defined with its own specific set of symptoms. This is supposed to be the psoric and sycotic combination but is not wholly accepted by all homeopaths, despite its obvious relationship to current disharmonies.

The "experts" feel that all miasms are incorporated within the primary three, as defined by Hahnemann, and no additional miasms are necessary. Although society continues to evolve, (or in some cases regress), it would appear that any new miasm discussion would combine two of the initial three in some fashion or another. We could have an AIDS miasm or a psychological miasm, but it is more a matter of semantics until we can define a new miasm in its own terms, rather than preexisting ones.

The Tubercular predisposition would seem to fit the picture of a new miasm, with its uniqueness and ancient history. Tuberculosis has been detected in the skeletons of primitive man and perhaps is one of the first diseases discovered by mankind.

With each miasm, there is a corresponding nosode. A nosode is a remedy made specifically from diseased tissue, such as Tuberculinum, which is pus from a pulmonary tubercular abscess. Obviously, these nosodes are potentized to eliminate toxicity and create a true homeopathic remedy.

Each miasm has its own unique presentation and symptom picture. In addition to the nosode which relates to the miasm, many remedies strongly interact well with certain miasmatic tendencies. Some even cover more than one miasm and are often polycrests with broad symptom pictures. The following provides some insight into the different miasms, their pictures, symptoms and related remedies.

Miasms: An Inherited Tendency

Psora

Psora was the first miasm Hahnemann described and used, and being as it is the underlying miasm to all chronic conditions, pathology and other miasms, it will be our first stop on the miasmatic trail.

Hahnemann felt that psora, or scabies, was like "original sin". It is the cause for all subsequent disorders, being the most "ancient, universal and destructive" disease known to mankind. Each individual carries the psoric miasm and it's rarely eliminated, although with the correct choice of homeopathic remedy, a balance can be established.

The main focus of the psoric miasm is the skin and it developed as a result of suppression of the "itch", or scabies infection. Deficiency is the key term used to explain psora and it encompasses insufficiency, inhibition and inability or lack.

Roger Morrison describes the nosode Psorinum as having a poverty consciousness, and this accurately reflects the feeling of lack for the entire psoric tendency.

Most psoric disorders relate to a functional disharmony rather than a structural one, meaning that the pathology produces imbalance on the levels of sensation. This can be seen as itching, burning of the skin, inflammation, allergies, hypersensitivity or congestion. Hyperactivity is also a component.

To fully understand this miasm, lets review the indications, symptoms, limitations and development.

As mentioned above, the miasm developed from suppressed scabies, but the original infestation came from fluid in the vesicles or pustules, which were transferred by contact with the skin. This form of physical contact established entry into the skin of a second individual by the "itch mite." For several days after contact, there is no appearance of an itch or eruption.

During this time, the "mite" begins to infest the entire organism and establish its stronghold. Outward manifestation begins in the form of eruptions and itching at the original place of contact. If suppressed by medications or ointments, the "mite" is driven inward and becomes dormant.

This dormancy period can be triggered or awakened by any number of traumas or causes, effecting not only the physical level but the emotional and mental levels as well. Suppressed psora strongly impacts the nervous system, which directly connects to the hypersensitivity and hyperactivity previously described.

The following provides some of the indications and symptoms related to psora:

Restless, hurried and nervous.

Selfish.

Deceitful and secretive, may lack morals.

Prefers solitude and isolation.

Can be timid or slow of mind.

Past or present history of skin disharmony; burning sensations.

Inability to complete ideas.

Inhibited nature.

Weakness and easily fatigued.

Low self-esteem.

Redness and dryness of mucus membranes.

Helplessness and self-reproach.

Lack of vital heat.

Feels better with any type of discharge.

Pains are of a neuralgic type, sore and bruised feeling.

"Hypo" conditions, such as hypothyroid, hypotension.

Feels worse standing.

Constipation.

A "burnt" taste in the mouth.

Hoards or saves many things.

Fears of failure or being totally alone.

Poor memory.

Other symptoms are better when skin disharmony reappears.

Poor metabolism, often slow; overweight.

Manifestation of illness around the age of 40.

Desires sweet, salty, fried and spicy foods; aversion to milk.

Better: Lying down, summer, warmth, activity, discharges.

Worse: winter, cold, standing, during sleep.

Some specific psoric remedies, relating to the above symptoms and indications:

Arsenicum Album: burning sensations, restless.

Arsenicum Iodatum: a warm blooded Arsenicum Album

Apis: burning, itching, stinging sensations.

Hepar Sulf: hypersensitive and irritable.

Lachesis: better after discharges begin.

Lycopodium: insecure, weak, selfish, timid and sensitive.

Natrum Mur: closed, prefers solitude, allergies and loves salt.

Nitric Acid: hypersensitive, irritable, negative, anxious.

Psorinum: chilly, anxious, hopeless, truly poverty conscious.

Selenium: despair, irritability, theorizes, skin disharmony.

Sepia: fatigue, low esteem, constipation, irritable.

Sulphur: worse standing, thinker, burning sensations.

Zincum: oversensitive, irritable, restless and complains.

Consider: *Aloe; Calcarea Carb, Phos, Sil and Sulf; Clematis; Graphites; Mezerium; Petroleum; Sarsparilla; Stannum.*

Psora's limiting factors relate to the specific tendencies of "lack". The overall insufficiency, affecting all spheres, limits well-being, growth, recovery, career and motivation. These limitations extend to concentration abilities, apathy and indifference, fears, anxieties and depression. The psoric individual is full of ideas, but without the mental, emotional or physical resources to bring them to fruition.

Practically every aspect of expression is limited within the Psoric predisposition. That tendency even relates to the strong desire for solitude which is a large component of this miasm. The need to be alone stems from an inability to relate to others and an inner sense of worthlessness. They prefer to dwell in isolation for safety, thus limiting their fear of being emotionally hurt.

Psora also weaves its trail into the sycotic miasm, bringing with it various skin ailments, most notably growths such as warts and tumors.

Sycosis

The Sycotic miasm developed from suppressed gonorrhea or as described in past medical history as "fig wart" disease. The term is derived from the appearance of the diseased growth which resembled a fig. This miasm represents the pathological condition of excessiveness, including overabundance of mucus and various growths.

It evolved when doctors felt the need to remove these growths by cutting or burning them off. The external lesion or growth was eliminated but internal development was established creating a secondary disharmony. This secondary action was not always manifested immediately, often taking years before distinct symptoms arose.

Sycosis is carried genetically to succeeding generations and not necessarily with the appearance of growths or warts. Often it can be recognized in the vertical ridges of the nails or in psychological inclinations.

Dr. Burnett discovered that a strong similarity exists between the sycotic symptom picture and repeated pox vaccinations. Although small pox vaccinations have been eliminated, ill effects continue to surface in genetic pictures due to the initial impact it created on the system. A detailed discussion on vaccinations will come in a later chapter.

Medorrhinum is the corresponding nosode to the sycotic miasm and is not well represented in *Kent's Repertory*, although it is presented well in the three most recent ones. Without knowing its general indications, a homeopath would rarely come to prescribe Medorrhinum from use of *Kents'*

Repertory alone. It is prepared from the discharge of an untreated case of gonorrhea, containing both bacteria and human tissue. The toxicity is removed by homeopathic potentization.

To better comprehend the Sycotic miasm, the following symptoms provide a picture of the typical case:

Proliferation of tissue, tumors, growths.

Suspiciousness.

Restless and hyperactive.

Cruel.

Poor memory for recent events.

Irritability with fits of anger.

Secretive.

Suicidal tendencies or thoughts of destruction.

Quarrelsome.

Deceitful.

Selfish.

Forgets words or loses train of thought.

Self-reproach or condemnation.

Past shame or humiliation.

Low self-esteem.

Mental conditions are better with growth of warts.

Mischievous predisposition.

Vertigo or dizziness.

Headaches which are worse at night or with exertion.

Chronic nasal discharges; hayfever.

Loss of smell.

Moles.

Fishy taste or odor.

Predisposition to bronchitis and teasing coughs.

Asthma.

Joint pains from gout.

Herpes and zoster.

Menstrual pains.

Leucorrhea.

Pelvic Inflammatory Disease.

Appendicitis.
Prostate enlargement.
Ringworm.
Worse any barometric changes.
High blood pressure.
Excess perspiration with a fishy odor.
Desires: salt, fatty meat, seasoned foods, peppers, beer.
Aversions: milk, wine, spices.
Worse: damp, cold, rainy seasons, rest, humidity, heat.
Better: dry atmosphere, movement or activity, winter.
Remedies which strongly relate to the sycotic miasm are:
Argentum Metallicum: pains appear suddenly; vertigo.
Kali Iodatum: irritable and cruel; hayfever; asthma; arthritis.
Kali Sulf: low confidence; irritability; headaches; asthma.
Lycopodium: low esteem; perspiration; leucorrhea; herpes.
Medorrhinum: herpes; chronic discharges; excess/extremes.
Natrum Sulf: gonorrhea; suicidal; mental dullness; warts.
Nitric Acid: negative, irritable, cursing; herpes; vaginitis.
Radium Brom: joints; irritability; moles; gout; tickling cough.
Sepia: irritable; mental dullness; PMS; fishy odor; herpes.
Staphysagria: shame; self-reproach; low confidence; anger.
Tarantula: deceitful; destructive; tumors; restless/hyper.
Thuja: feels worthless; herpes; warts; secretive; gonorrhea.
Consider: *Arsenicum album and Iodatum; Mezerum; Natrum Mur; Psorinum; Pyrogenium; Lachesis; Sarsparilla; Silica.*
On the sexual sphere there are many disturbances observed through disharmonies relating to the sexual organs. Frequently, the sexual desire is quite strong, with the exception of Sepia. The resulting increased desires may manifest

in pelvic inflammatory disease, herpes, leucorrhea, cystitis, vaginitis, ovarian tumors, cysts and vaginal warts.

The nosode Medorrhinum has often been described as the sex, drugs and rock and roll remedy, especially when excess is involved. Perhaps this is indicative of the 1970's free love lifestyle. Under any circumstance, the totality is taken into consideration for every remedy chosen, and this includes the cause of any subsequent diseased state.

General metabolism is also effected by this miasm—a form of in-coordination of the body's ability to assimilate energy. From this inability comes pituitary malfunction such as dwarfism or cretinism. There can be deficient growth on all levels, including both mental and physical aspects.

Cancer may also be a by-product of this miasm, considering the inclination toward growths, cysts and tumors. Also, the color yellow is strongly associated with the Sycotic miasm, which includes freckles, liver spots and jaundice.

Keep in mind that all disease can be associated with the later stages of any one of the miasms, simply as a result of overall disharmony and disfunction of the system as a whole. In this regard, a miasm is not the cause but more a reflection of the organisms disintegration.

Syphilitic

The third chronic miasm described by Hahnemann stems from the suppression of syphilis, another venereal disease. Infection stems from sexual intercourse where a pustule arises anywhere from 7 to 14 days after contact. If left uncured, it remains throughout the lifetime, growing over the years and precluding any additional symptoms from arising. If removed or suppressed in any manner, secondary symptoms manifest on deeper levels.

Syphilinum is the nosode for this miasm and mirrors its many aspects. Destruction is the key element, although rarely violent in nature. It's more of a wearing away action along the lines of osteoporosis. This destructive tendency infiltrates

Homeopathic Vibrations

the mental, emotional and physical make-up of the system causing degeneration on each level.

In the final stages of the miasm, violence and destruction erupt, both outwardly and inwardly. In other words, either homicide or suicide.

The syphylitic miasm is often considered the most destructive of all, as it can destroy the vital force in its degenerative action. It creates imbalance and disharmony, diminishing equilibrium in the system. Syphilis affects the vital organs in the secondary or suppressed stages, more so than either of the other miasms.

Some of the major characteristics include:

Depression and sadness.
Desires solitude.
Suicidal predisposition.
Secretive, even about their own pains.
Mental dullness.
Forgetful.
Perversion/wicked.
Compulsive.
Rigid and fixed ideas.
Desire to kill.
Pessimistic.
Hair oily and greasy.
Head and ears are large.
Loss of smell.
Poor vision.
Teeth not symmetric.
Metallic taste in mouth.
Wrinkled, old appearance.
Rough skin.
Nails are spoon shaped and thin.
Many bone pains.
Ulcers of the skin.
Distortions of the anatomy.
Low sexual desire.

Desires: stimulants, smoking, cold food, indigestible things, sour.

Aversions: meat, animal foods.

Better: sunrise, change of position, temperate climate, cold.

Worse: night, seashore, warmth, summer, night sweats.

Listed below are some remedies well suited to the syphilitic miasm:

Aurum: depressed, suicidal, pains worse at night; aversion meat.

Fluoric Acid: isolated, materialistic, indifferent, weak nails.

Hepar: sensitive, irritable, suicidal, offensive odors, skin ulcers.

Kali Iodatum: harsh temper, cruel, worse at night, syphilis.

Kali Sulf: depressed, low esteem, warm blooded, bone pains.

Lachesis: suspicious, jealous, introverted, alcoholism, hot.

Mercurius: instability, low confidence, sensitive, perspiration high.

Nitric Acid: oversensitive, selfish, fearful, angry, chilly, curses.

Phytolacca: shameless; mastitis; sore throat; restless; soreness.

Silica: low esteem, lacks stamina, constipation, yeilding, sensitive.

Stillingia: chronic fatigue, cough after flu; gloom; dullness; dry.

Syphilinum: dread of night, compulsive; chilly; destructive; pains.

Consider: *Arsenicum Alb; Calcarea Ars; Conium; Iodatum; Ledum; Lycopodium; Mercury's; Phosphorus; Phosphoric acid; Staphysagria.*

The depression of the syphilitic miasm is profound, yet the emotion is frequently kept a secret and upon suicide, friends or co-workers might indicate they had no idea of the despair. There is also a deep-seated dishonesty and deceit, which comes from their inner feeling of worthlessness. They will lie and cheat to get ahead or have others feel sorry for them. It provides a sense of power over others which is typical of their malicious and destructive manner.

When there is a family or past history of abortions, heart problems, insanity, cancer, tuberculosis, suicide or sterility, the syphylitic miasm is an underlying current. Syphylitic predispositions or suppressions will manifest around the age of 40, either on the physical, emotional or mental level.

There is a plethora of skin ailments, including excema, psoriasis, ulcerations, offensive bloody or pus filled discharges and gangrene. Rarely though, is itching associated with these maladies. Most of the natural discharges cause an aggravation, unlike psoric individuals who feel better with such discharges.

Tuberculin

It was stated earlier that the tubercular miasm creates confusion in the homeopathic community as it is often considered a combination of the Psora and Syphilitic miasms. The truth may fall somewhere in the middle, but tuberculosis appears to be distinct enough to have specifically related symptoms and characteristics. As mentioned, all of the miasms interrelate in some fashion or another, so cross symptoms arise frequently.

It was in the 1600's that tuberculosis was first labeled, although its destruction was established long before its diagnosis. The causative organism is mycobacteria which is a highly contagious airborne pathogen. Symptoms include formation of tubercles (small tissue nodules), inflammation and caseous necrosis (tissues which become soft, dry and curdled). The active disease has an incubation period of one to two years after infection. Although it primarily focuses on the respiratory system, it can affect any part of the body, including the lymph system, bones, muscles and joints.

Tuberculinum is the nosode for this miasm yet it reflects its own unique picture and distinguishing symptoms. The individual is anxious, averse to most mental work, complaining, possibly depressed and irritable with a strong desire for travel and change. Physically, there is an overall fatigue, with chilliness, a tendency to catch colds easily, poor circulation, desire for open air, emaciation and insomnia with frightful dreams.

Generally, a miasm is partially defined by the symptoms contained within its nosode and the Tuberculin miasm follows this pattern. The miasmatic literature is not as extensive as with preceding miasms nor as clearly defined. One word descriptions used with each of the miasms, such as "lack" for psora and "growths" for the sycotic, are not as obvious for the Tuberculin and Cancer miasms.

Nonetheless, the Tuberculin miasm seems to reflect "a wasting away" and "dissatisfaction" as two of its stronger characteristics. Most everything in this miasm seems to relate to tuberculosis, with the exception of the mentals.
The symptoms are as follows:
Slow mental comprehension.
Lack of tolerance.
Dissatisfied with everything.
Capricious and changeable moods and attitudes.
Changes places, jobs and relationships frequently.
Depression without hopelessness.
Indifference.
Inability to concentrate.
Uncontrollable passions.
Fear of dogs.
Irritable.
Quarrelsome.
Angry.
Carelessness.
Weakness with fatigue.
Glands are affected.
Desires foods which cause disharmony.
Headaches which are periodic.

Allergies and hay fever.

Symptoms often are better with a natural discharge.

Offensive odors.

Astigmatism and photophobia.

Cheesy ear discharges.

Face flushes easily with circumscribed spots.

Ulcers in the mouth.

Asthma, tuberculosis, coughs.

Quick response to weather changes.

Worms.

Joint problems.

Eczema, herpes, impetigo.

Varicose veins.

Freckles.

Desires: indigestible things, salts, fats, tobacco, grease, potatoes.

Aversions: meat, fat of meat.

Better: day time, dry, open air.

Worse: night, thunderstorms, greasy foods.

Listed below are some possible remedies for the Tubercular miasm:

Arsenicum Iodatum: allergies, asthma, eczema, restlessness.

Bacillinum: depressed, irritable, takes colds easily, humid asthma.

Baryta Carb: better open air, ulcers mouth, wasting away, glands.

Calcarea Carb: despair of recovery, weakness, allergies, fear dogs.

Calcarea Phos: love travel, irritable, complaining, fatigue, allergy.

Hepar: irritable, oversensitive, anxious, chilly, glandular swelling.

Iodum: hurried, changeable, emaciation, fatigue, hay fever, asthma.

Lycopodium: depression, low esteem, fatigue, freckles, skin.

Natrum Sulf: asthma, photophobia, worse night, eczema, allergies.

Phosphorus: fearful, anxious, freckles, loves travel, sensitive.

Sepia: irritable, chilly, indifferent, overwhelmed, fatigue, depressed.

Silica: lack stamina, chilly, failure to thrive, anxious, head sweats.

Stannum: depletion and weakness, headaches, poor respiration.

Thuja: depression, chilly, headaches, secretive, herpes, allergies.

Tuberculinum: desires travel, tuberculosis, irritable, allergies.

Zincum: complaining, restless, irritable, oversensitive, insomnia.

Consider: *Kali's, Hydrastis, Pulsatilla, Spongia, Sulphur, Tarantula, Nitric Acid, Carcinosin, Carbo Animalis, Sanicula Aqua.*

Children's hyperactivity is another component of the Tubercular miasm and this includes ADD (attention deficit disorders). "Problem children" also fit the symptom picture. Often though, there may be destructive and malicious tendencies, either for others or for the children themselves. Head banging, screaming, striking, biting and throwing things are additional behavior disorders.

On the adult level, there is a more "cosmopolitan" nature, a desire for change and travel that cannot be fulfilled. Mental alertness does not coincide with the physical debility and fatigue. Despite eating well, there can be a tendency toward emaciation and thinness.

There may be a history of tuberculosis in the family or even allergies, especially to cats. Ringworm or worms may be a part of the family history as well. Diarrhea can be chronic, along with early or prolonged bedwetting.

The fingernails have white spots, are thin, brittle, break and split easily and are wavy or stained. One rather unique aspect is the caved in chest area, called a "pigeon chest". The hair is thin and dry. Bleeding from the nose or rectum is another symptom of this miasm.

With the Psoric and the Syphylitic potential within the Tubercular, there is a common thread of symptoms covering both of these miasms. It should be noted that Tuberculosis can be either inherited or acquired and that with proper remedy selection, eliminated.

A disease of this nature can be life-threatening and care should be taken in avoiding aggravations or overstimulation by giving too high of a potency.

Tuberculosis seems to be on the rise again, with a new and pervasive strain which allopathic drugs have had difficulty in eliminating or preventing. Homeopathy will always look to the patient not the label or the symptoms, so new strains will be no different from the older ones against its effectiveness.

Cancer

Cancer is a malignant cellular tumor, divided into two distinct categories, carcinoma (malignant growth of epithelial cells) and sarcoma (a malignancy which develops from connective tissue of the bone, muscle or tendons).

Various causes, including environmental, chemical, emotional, dietary and inherited predispositions have contributed to malignant growths. The development and specific cause of these malignancies is not entirely clear, but it appears that there is often more than one factor involved in its spread.

As the immune system is weakened, from any of the above or additional causes, its ability to ward off illness and tumors diminishes. The human body and a castle have something in common. Both have systems of protection. The body has an immune system while a castle has a moat. When the moat is filled with protective water or creatures, the castle remains strong and guarded. Should the moat become weak or lose its water, the castle is more susceptible to an invasion.

The body is inundated with germ and bacteria warfare every second of the day. Should susceptibility be greater than normal due to poor diet, stress, environment, lack of exercise or poor hygiene, microorganisms overcome the immune system. Sensitivities can be generated from an overreaction to the weather, household cleaners or any number of sources. Continued sensitivity over a long period of time further weakens the immune system, triggering a greater susceptibility to a cancerous predisposition.

Every individual has some inherited inclination to cancer, but through proper diet, exercise and moderation, the subsequent tendency is frequently limited. Then there are the individuals who have no regard for lifestyle and moderation and seem to live without illness or disease. Always remember to account for the exception to the general rule.

The Cancer miasm is an interrelated story, reflecting a predisposition to growths of all types, including malignant ones. The underlying aspect coincides with a diminished immune system in conjunction with some form of stimulus which triggers growth of the malignant cells. Destructive cells can be spread by various means, such as needles, blood, organ metastasis and perhaps saliva or vaginal secretions.

As mentioned previously, growths are a primary aspect of the Cancer miasm and they take the form of warts, moles, birthmarks, tumors, cysts and herpetic eruptions. Of all the miasms and related nosodes, this particular one seems to be the softest in relation to the emotions. There does not seem to be the destructiveness, maliciousness or deep depression of the others.

The nosode, Carcinosin, helps to define the miasm, especially since this miasm is a combination of the psoric and sycotic predispositions. Carcinosin is often passionate, obsessive, fastidious, sympathetic, sensitive and full of worries.

Physically, there is constipation, asthma or respiratory problems, strong and early sexual propensities, moles on the face, neck and back, skin disharmonies, insomnia and a history of cancer or diabetes in the family.

Symptom indications for the cancer miasm and for cancer include:

Insomnia.

Family history of cancer, diabetes or tuberculosis.

Early history of disease (whooping cough, asthma, mononucleosis).

Malignant growths.

Moles, warts or other growths.

Skin or mouth ulcerations which do not heal.

Pains which have no cause.

Unusual lumps.

Hoarseness, constant need to clear throat.

Ongoing digestive problems, without appetite.

Relentless low-grade fevers.

Degenerative disharmonies of all types.

Unusual or continuous bleeding.

Chronic constipation with swelling of lower extremities.

Changing color of warts or moles.

Anxieties and fears which increase without cause.

A feeling of emotional foreboding.

Feeling worse at night and when alone.

Exhaustion and fatigue.

Better when with family and friends.

In need of support and nurturing.

The symptom picture for the Cancer miasm is not as extensive as the others, yet symptoms are commonly found in the disease state itself. As is the case with the Tubercular miasm, when well-chosen remedies fail to act in accordance with typical homeopathic standards, Carcinosin may assist in clearing the case. Cancer associated remedies are listed on the following page:

Argentricum Nit: fears, ulcerations, digestive problems, fatigue.

Arsenicum Alb: skin disharmonies, fears, worse alone, bleeding.

Aurum: suicidal, abandonment, fearful, pains at night, fibroids.

Bromium: glandular swelling, hoarseness, asthma, tumors.

Calcarea Ars: anxieties, colitis, pains, fatigue, fears, growths.

Carbo Animalis: swelling of glands, weakness, fibroids, pains.

Carcinosin: insomnia, constipation, history of mononucleosis, cysts, fatigue.

Chelidonium: malignancies, liver and digestive problems.

Echinacea: ulcerations, sores, pains, fatigue, lymphatic swellings.

Hydrastis: depression, ulcers, stomach cancer, indigestion.

Iodum: restless, compulsive, better with activities, asthma.

Kreosotum: cysts, tumors, bleeding, gastritis, hoarseness, coughs.

Lachesis: anxieties, asthma, colitis, ovarian cysts, tumors.

Nitric Acid: negative, anxious, herpes, ulcers, bleeding, warts.

Phosphorus: fearful, anxious, fibroids, ulcers, hoarseness, bleeding.

Phytolacca: worse night, tumors, fibroids, pains, bleeding.

Scirrhinum: breast cancer, tumors, cysts, glandular hardness.

Consider: *Alumina, Calcarea Carb, Calcarea Sulf, Cadmium Sulf, Bufo, China, Graphites, Carbo Veg, Kali Ars, Mercurius Sol, Ignacia, Lycopodium, Natrum Mur, Natrum Carb, Thuja, Sulphur, Zincum.*

Cancer's impact on society has been remarkable. The degeneration of the immune system and its subsequent inability to overcome invasion has allowed this disease to proliferate and create destruction. Working with homeopathy in the classical sense (one remedy at a time and the symptom totality), cure and elimination can become common place. Succeeding generations will have the opportunity to reduce malignancies, strengthen the immune system and establish balance throughout the system.

Vaccinations can play a part in weakening the immune system. Despite the attempt to eliminate disease, more often, vaccines alter the normal course of recovery.

Tri-miasmatic Remedies

Generally, working on the miasmatic levels is not the first choice of practicing homeopaths, at least not in the earlier stages of practice. Miasmatic understanding is difficult and requires experience and patience, especially with the possibility of more than one miasm within each individual.

The nosodes are used like all other remedies, but in choosing a nosode, the corresponding miasm is often present. From this association, additional miasmatic remedies can be reviewed to determine effectiveness on the presenting symptoms.

This is a backhanded approach to utilizing miasmatic theory and symptoms, but it works. By understanding certain remedies, such as Mercurius and Aurum, the practitioner will begin to understand the Syphylitic miasm. And when these remedies are used without result or cure, then the analogous nosode may often clear or even cure the case.

As discussed several times previously, *the most well-suited remedy*, whether a nosode or a related miasmatic remedy, *is chosen on the complete picture of the individual*, not just specific symptoms. Causative factors, history and personality are most determinative in remedy selection.

Miasmatic tendencies and symptoms often overlap causing even greater confusion. Look to the current or presenting miasm, or the one creating the most disharmony and work specifically with it. Then the underlying miasm becomes clearer.

For instance, with Psoric and Sycotic aspects, first clear the Psoric as much as possible, then the Sycotic, then return to the Psoric. Obviously, this is only true if the Psoric is the first and strongest presenting symptom picture. Psora is the mother and father of all subsequent miasmatic pictures and is often the last miasm before cure.

Should there be a presentation of all three miasms in the same individual, which is not all that infrequent, the above still applies. It may take several years to accomplish balance and healing, but in considering the longevity of the disharmony, two or three years are insignificant. Especially, when the symptoms diminish and health improves over that period.

The following remedies have been proven valuable for all three primary miasms, covering aspects of each in some fashion or another: They are called Tri-miasmatic.

Aurum
Argentum Metallicum
Bascilinum
Calcarea's
Carcinosin
Iodum
Lycopodium
Mercurius
Nitric Acid
Phytolacca
Psorinum
Staphysagria
Sulphur
Thuja
Tuberculinum

The study of miasms can be both exciting and difficult. Ultimately, it is really just another tool to have available in understanding a person's disharmony. When a remedy fails to hold or provide cure, then consider the miasmatic predisposition or the miasmatic nosode. A miasm may well be the underlying condition that prevents action of a remedy. Always consider this factor when several remedies should have worked, yet there was little success.

If those remedies were within the same miasm, such as the Aurum and Mercurius mentioned above, then evaluate the Syphlitic tendency and review Syphlinum as a next step. Even in that situation, the nosode must fit the person's totality.

Given that miasms are frequently overlooked in evaluation and analysis, this information may help unlock difficult and hard to clear cases, opening the way for guiding symptoms and an effective remedy. There are times when a nosode will both clear and cure, but more often, a follow-up remedy is needed to complete the action of the nosode.

Hahnemann's Organon has some wonderful information on the miasms and their relationship with disease and chronic disharmonies. A more detailed study of the Organon follows this chapter in order to get a full picture of the information Hahnemann provided.

It would seem more appropriate to have discussed this material at an earlier point, but the Organon is often difficult, repetitious and overwhelming to someone just beginning to delve into the principles and philosophies of homeopathy. Reading it at any stage is not easy, but with the underlying precepts and examples previously provided, it becomes less so.

Each paragraph or aphorism builds upon the preceding one, yet to analyze each one in depth before reading the Organon would be an injustice to Hahnemann's efforts.

Chapter Twelve

The Organon: Hahnemann's Principles of Healing

As briefly mentioned in prior Chapters, the Organon is the work upon which homeopathy is based. Six separate editions were written over Hahnemann's lifetime. The last was not published until decades after his death. As with all books of this stature, controversy surrounded the publication of each of the Organon's, from the first to the sixth edition.

In the beginning, Hahnemann's work was scoffed at and ridiculed because it did not correspond with current medical thinking. With time, experience and results came credibility and acceptance, even with the ruling elite. By the time the sixth edition was published, it was the homeopaths who refused to accept some of the newer principles and ideas that Hahnemann put forth.

This was mostly the result of Hahnemann's almost exclusive use of LM potencies in the later years of his life and his inclusion of the LM methods in the sixth edition. He determined that the LM potency, a dilution of a 3c in 500 drops of water, eliminated or reduced aggravations, especially for sensitive individuals.

Homeopaths had good success with c and x potencies and were reluctant to attempt the use of LM potencies, which had questionable beginnings. The question arose as to who actually wrote about the LM's. Notes were found in the margins of the fifth edition of the Organon while it was not clear who wrote them. With the questions came doubts. Since the fifth edition philosophies and potencies were effectively working, many set the sixth edition aside as the meandering of an old man or the writings of his wife, Melanie.

Others began using the newer potencies with greater success and fewer aggravations, establishing its foothold in the homeopathic community. Today, all three types of potencies are used, each in their own manner and each with effectiveness for specific circumstances.

There are 291 paragraphs or aphorisms in the sixth edition. They are broken down into two distinct parts: theory and practicum. The first 70 aphorisms relate to the theoretical components and the remainder with practical ones.

It is impossible to give a complete detailed description of each paragraph of the Organon, or for that matter one that does justice to Hahnemann's incredible work, but the following may provide some insight into their meaning.

Paragraphs 5 through 18 center around the knowledge of disease, its causes, types, history, the need for removal and the means to accomplish it; he defines both health and disease, influences upon disease, results of various influences, an interconnection of disease and the organism, a manifestation of symptoms and the summation of all symptoms toward one solution—a remedy.

Paragraphs 19 through 27 deal with the knowledge of medicines, their power to alter a state of ill health, their power to provide a proving by dosing a healthy individual, their curative principles, their similarities to a diseased state, aggravations from dosing, their ability to create an artificial state in a healthy person, the permanent removal of symptoms with the medicines, the theory of that removal, their strength and the superiority of the medicine to specific symptoms.

Paragraphs 28 through 70 reflect the choice of the remedy along with its administration. Number 70 specifically summarizes these aphorisms by discussing the totality of symptoms, the Law of Similars, suitable doses, a remedy's ability to overpower disease, the only true possible means of cure (homeopathy), extinguishing disease in a permanent fashion, irritations to the vital force and an explanation of the life principle.

The Aphorisms relating to the practical aspects of homeopathy begin with paragraphs 71 through 100 and deal directly with how a practitioner can determine what is important in casetaking. These paragraphs discuss acute and chronic disease and provide an explanation of vital energy and its components. The miasms are mentioned in relation to the chronic disharmonies as predisposed tendencies of the organism and its inability to fully recover from interrelated diseases.

Hahnemann indicates that precise casetaking with particular detail and in spontaneous fashion, assists in the selection of the best-suited remedy for the most effective results. All symptoms are taken in their totality with modalities and time references as guiding characteristics of the presenting picture. Emotional disposition and temperament are given greater weight when obtained voluntarily, but given significant weight under all circumstances.

Paragraphs 100 through 105 continue with the casetaking process and give further insight into the specifics of observation and the totality of distinguishing symptoms.

The next aphorisms, numbered 105 through 145, shed light on how to acquire knowledge of the curative aspects of the remedies and how they can be used to cure. In studying the remedies, the pathogenic effects are of greater importance, particularly the symptoms and alterations of health that each is capable of producing in a healthy person. The only way to ascertain these effects is through the provings. By reading the provings, a student will get a glimpse of the underlying picture of each remedy and its essence or causative aspects.

Peculiar or unusual symptom pictures of the remedies can provide an effective study guide for each remedy. Paragraphs 105 through 145 deliberately and accurately describe the nature of a proving. Within each specific description comes the understanding of cure and how they can be used to bring about that cure.

Paragraphs 146 through 285 provide information on the most effective means for using remedies in an effort to eliminate disease and establish permanent cure.

Provings and aggravations are discussed in these aphorisms, along with minor acute and chronic disease states, minimum dosing, disturbance and unobserved symptom pictures during a disharmony, specific and necessary remedy reactions (paragraph 165), remedy selection and one-sided diseases which obscure a full symptom presentation.

The need for surgery in certain instances is described in paragraph 186. Causative factors are addressed, as is totality of the symptom picture, complete investigation of all causes, the vital force and its relationship to disharmony and health, inquiries into sexually transmitted diseases, history taking (aphorism 208), the interconnection of mental, emotional and physical symptoms, psora as underlying foundation for all chronic or acute disease and intermittent states of disharmony.

Beginning with paragraph 246, Hahnemann discusses the procedure for employing the remedies and the regimen to be observed during their use. Included is potentization, succussions, dosing, intervals between dosing, neutralization of aggravations, amelioration of symptoms, observations, obstacles to cure, purity of the medicines, preparation of the medicines, LM potencies (Aphorism 270), water dilutions, single dosing, sensitivities, placebos and the smallest doses.

Alternative therapeutic agents are mentioned in the concluding paragraphs, 286 through 291. These agents, which are not specifically homeopathic medicines, include magnetism, electricity, hypnotism, massage and baths.

There are some distinct changes and differences between the fifth and sixth edition of the Organon. The sixth edition contains rewritten paragraphs, deletions, additions, new processes and possibly unauthorized corrections.

The Organon: Hahnemann's Principles of Healing

The final Organon was published in 1921, almost eighty years after Hahnemann's death. There are three fewer aphorisms than in the fifth edition. Also, the sixth edition discussed certain external applications of medicines, which were discouraged in earlier versions.

The Organon is the true foundation of homeopathy but not frequently read or understood. Possibly because it was repetitious and contained unique material that was beyond Hahnemann's time. Maybe because it is just not an easy book to read. It is interesting to note that some of the precepts and theories precede much of what is currently accepted in microbiology.

The Organon is a book worth reading and one that contains information of significant value in a society that seeks self-responsibility for health and healing.

Chapter Thirteen

Vaccinations: A Review

How does the vaccination theory relate to homeopathy? In the truest sense, it does not. But with respect to possible causes of disharmony, it has a strong relationship. Miasms were discussed in a previous chapter, along with miasmatic predispositions and interrelated causes for succeeding generational disharmonies.

Vaccinations may very well have the same effect, not only upon the generations receiving them, but on subsequent generations. We are affected by vaccines on the cellular level and any mutation on this level is passed on to children.

Most vaccines contain carbolic acid, formaldehyde, mercury, aluminum phosphate and acetone as preservatives. Regardless of the intent and the miniscule amount, these agents affect the system, and not always as intended.

The federal government has a program which compensates the families of children who have adverse or debilitating reactions to a vaccine. This program is funded in the hundred's of millions of dollars, paying millions each year to children disabled from vaccinations. Yet both the government and doctors continue to profess the safety of and the continued need for disabling vaccines.

Numerous reports and studies have found a definite causative relationship to various illnesses stemming from vaccinations. They range from brain damage to seizures to attention deficit disorders. There are also less damaging disorders like fevers, rashes, pains, emotional distress and irritability.

Do we need to be vaccinated? Probably not. Polio was already on the decline when vaccinations began in the United States. Countries like England had no vaccine mandates and survived the outbreak. There is currently no diphtheria in the United States, yet we continue to vaccinate for this disease at the age of eight weeks, along with pertussin and tetanus. It is true that pertussis can be fatal in children before the age of one, but what is not mentioned is the fact that the vaccine can contribute to a greater susceptibility to the disease.

Why are we vaccinated? Because the medical and pharmaceutical communities are convinced that they are an effective means of preventing illness. This is not based solely on an altruistic mindset, but as much on an economic one. Pharmacies make money from producing the vaccine and after having spent enormous sums to develop them, they seek a return on their investment. The government has also been convinced of this theory. Why then does the government need a multimillion dollar fund to assist those who are disabled by the vaccines if they are so safe?

Are the long-term effects of vaccinations known? No. Our society labors under the delusion that if the government, pharmacies, and doctors say that a vaccine is potentially safe, then it must be safe. Of all the vaccines given, both to infants and adults alike, only 7 percent had no side effects. These side effects can produce a wide range of disharmonies and disabilities.

What exactly is a vaccine? It is a preparation of specific microorganisms (viruses, germs, bacteria) that may or may not be alive. These organisms are injected into the body in an attempt to prevent disease. The hoped for result is a build-up of immunity to the disease state, without additional ill effects.

It has been discovered that the injections can weaken the immune system so that greater susceptibility arises, not only to the specific disease itself but to other illnesses as well. The "other" disharmonies are the greater concern, simply because the system is often incapable of reestablishing its immunities to prevent attacks from unknown microorganisms.

Many of the required vaccines relate to childhood illnesses which are not often life-threatening, such as measles, mumps, chicken pox and even German measles or rubella. Some of

Vaccinations: A Review

the vaccines are for diseased states that are rare or nonexistent, with current outbreaks arising from the vaccines themselves, such as polio and diphtheria.

Three specific vaccines for pertussin, tetanus and hepatitis, may be as dangerous as the diseases they inoculate against. Of the three, the tetanus vaccine is the least damaging. Any long-term ill effects from the hepatitis vaccine are unknown. Tetanus usually comes from a puncture wound which allows a neurotoxin spore to enter the body causing muscle and respiratory spasms, lockjaw and contraction of the muscles. After a puncture wound of any type, a tetanus shot is usually given, even if one has been recently administered.

Tetanus is dangerous and can be fatal, but by allowing the blood to flow fully after the wound, the risk of tetanus is diminished. There are also several homeopathic remedies that can be administered to help prevent toxicity. These will be discussed shortly. It is best to err on the side of caution and get the tetanus vaccine in the event any question should arise regarding a deep puncture wound.

The pertussin vaccine has been known to affect a minimum of 3 percent of the children vaccinated. Of this 3 percent, brain damage is the most common result. Each year about three million infants are eligible for the vaccine. Of this number, there are over 900 deaths, 11,000 cases of long-term brain damage, about 19,000 with significant neurological disorders and over 4,000 with convulsions or collapse. Safe?

In Europe, vaccinations are no longer mandatory. Through studies completed after the voluntary use of vaccines was implemented, it was discovered that the incidence of fatalities from whooping cough (pertussis) had fallen dramatically. The reverse had been expected after the drop in vaccinations. Canadian studies and research seem to concur with the European reports.

Where does homeopathy fit into this mix? Those not fully educated in the theory and principles of homeopathy, equate vaccinations with homeopathic procedures. On the surface, that may appear true, but in the end, *likes that cure likes* in accordance with homeopathic ideals, does not include live bacteria that are injected into defenseless human beings. Homeopathy uses minute doses of similar resonance, not identical substances, nor are live microorganisms used.

Homeopathy is a proven science, used to stimulate the immune system, not diminish it. There has never been a case where a homeopathic remedy has caused multiple sclerosis, attention deficit disorders (ADD), seizures, brain damage, systemic lupus, convulsions, sudden infant death syndrome (SIDS), chromosome mutations or epilepsy, such as is the case with use of vaccinations.

Most of us are born with the capacity to combat illness, developed from an inherited supply of antibodies. Mother's milk also stimulates the immune system to increase its supply of antibodies. This occurs naturally, without need for outside reinforcement or vaccinations. Artificial inoculations diminish this natural ability, without proven effectiveness, but with obvious risks and dangers.

The decision to vaccinate is a difficult one, often based on pressure from friends, family and doctors. There is a fear factor and an assumption that the vaccine is effective and safe. Read before you vaccinate. The final choice should come from knowledge and education, not fear or blind compliance.

Several books to read about this decision, include: *DPT: A Shot in the Dark* by Harris Coulter; *The Immunization Decision* by Randall Neustaedter; *Vaccines: Are They Really Safe* by Neil Miller. Also, there are excellent articles in *Mothering Magazine* available and they will compile them for you upon request.

Homeopathy has a great deal to offer as an alternative to standard procedures both as a preventive and as an accelerated aid for recovery. There are specific remedies made from the vaccines which are diluted to eliminate any toxicity and which may act as prophylactics. The word "may" is used because verification is not always possible. The antibodies cannot be located, but the results are just as effective.

To illustrate the idea behind prevention, there is a case about Dr. Hahnemann's use of Belladonna for a little girl in need of it. Shortly after prescribing the remedy an outbreak of scarlet fever arose in her community and specifically within her family. The child was the only one not to contract the disease. Hahnemann attributed the powerful result to the effects of the Belladonna for its preventive action and its ability to enhance the immune system.

The list below represents remedies in relation to illness. However, bear in mind that specific nosodes, such as tetanus for lock-jaw, do not have clear provings of effects or causes:

For Chicken Pox:
Varicella as the nosode and prophylactic.
Aconite for the early stages with rash.
Antimonium Crudum when there are pustules that itch from warmth.
Pulsatilla will have a measles like rash.
Rhus Tox has intense itching that burns; also swollen glands.
Consider: *Antimonum Tart, Carbo-V, Ledum, Mercurius, Sulphur, Thuja.*

For Diphtheria:
Diptherinum as the nosode and prophylactic.
Arsenicum Album has high temperature, exhaustion and restlessness.
Belladonna for burning heat, delirium and no thirst or toxicity.
Lachesis for intermittent fevers with hot perspiration and flushes.
Mercurius Cyanatus has great prostration, coldness and nausea.
Phytolacca for glandular swelling, heat, prostration and chills.

Consider: *China-A, Ignacia, Kali-I, Kreosotum, Rhus Tox.*

For German Measles:

Rubella as the prophylactic and the nosode.

Aconite will have the measle like rash.

Belladonna when there is alternating redness and paleness of skin.

Ferrum Phos for the early stages and cold like symptoms.

Pulsatilla has a lack of thirst, swelling, rash and is needy.

For Hepatitis:

Potentitized Hepatitis as the nosode and prophylactic.

Carduus Marianus for pain in liver region, constipation and jaundice.

Chelidonium craves hot drinks, has distended abdomen with jaundice.

China has colic type pains, gas and bloating; liver is swollen; fever.

Lycopodium for sensitive liver area, digestive problems and pains.

Consider: *Aconite, Arsenicum-A, Belladonna, Natrum Sulf, Nux Vomica.*

For Measles:

Morbillinum is the nosode and prophylactic.

Apis for redness, burning, swelling and fells worse any heat.

Bryonia when any motion makes the itch worse; painful eruptions.

Euphrasia for the earliest stages; symptoms begin with the eyes.

Gelsemium when skin is hot, dry and itchy; fatigue with fever.

Consider: *Aconite, Belladonna, Pulsatilla, Rhus Tox.*

For Mumps:

Parotidinum as prophylactic and the nosode.

Baryta Carb when glands swell and tonsils are inflamed.

Calcarea-C has swelling, stitching pains and difficult swallowing.

Jaborandi is worse in the afternoon, with swelling and dryness.

Mercurius has redness, swelling, excess saliva and burning.

Consider: *Aconite, Belladonna, Apis, Lachesis, Phytolacca, Rhus Tox, Pulsatilla.*

For Polio:

Poliomyelitis potentized as prophylactic and nosode.

Calcarea-C helps for rheumatoid pains, weakness and swelling.

Causticum has painful joints, paralysis, numbness and restless legs.

Gelsemium when there is loss of power and muscular control; weak.

Lathyrus has rigidity of legs. numbness, paralysis and trembling.

Consider: *Aconite, Plumbum, Rhus Tox.*

For Scarlet Fever:

Scarlatinum as both prophylactic and nosode.

Apis has rash after fever; thirst; light sweat and sleepiness; heat.

Belladonna for abrupt onset with vomiting fever and sore throat.

Mercurius when there is increased saliva, swelling and burning.

Rhus Tox for restlessness with fever and chills; trembling; rash.

Consider: *Arsenicum-A; Bryonia; Lachesis, Nitric Acid, Gelsemium, Sulph.*

For Small Pox:

Variolinum covers both the nosode and prophylactic.

Antimonium Tart has pustular eruptions with bluish-red marks.
Mercurius for constantly wet skin, eruptions and glandular swelling.
Natrum Mur has crusty eruptions that itch and burn; dryness.
Thuja is sensitive to touch and eruptions on covered parts.
Consider: *Antimonium-C, Apis, Arsenicum, Bryonia, Rhus Tox, Sulphur.*

For Tetanus:
Tetanus potentized as nosode and prophylactic.
Arnica for any wound or trauma.
Cicuta has a profound effect on the nervous system with paralysis.
Hypericum for any puncture wound with radiating or tingling pains.
Ledum for puncture wounds with coldness but worse warmth; twitch.
Consider: *Aconite, Belladonna, Causticum, Gelsemium, Nux Vomica.*

For Typhoid:
Typhoidinum as prophylactic and nosode.
Agaricus for sensitivity to cold air, intense heat in evening; sweat.
Baptisia has chills, pains, prostration, soreness and heat.
China covers intermittent fevers, chills, excess sweats and thirst.
Gelsemium has slow pulse, trembling, chills, heat and sweat.
Phosphoric Acid for profuse sweat, chills, stupor and low fever.
Consider: *Apis, Arsenicum, Belladonna, Bryonia, Ferrum Phos, Lachesis, Nitric Acid, Phosphorus, Rhus Tox, Sulphur, Veratrum-A, Zincum.*

Vaccinations: A Review

For Whooping Cough:

Pertussin as prophylactic and nosode.

Antimonum Tart has a rattling sound with little expectoration.

Cuprum covers suffocative coughs with spasms and constriction.

Drosera has a dry irritating cough with choking sensation; hoarse.

Kali Sulph for croupy type cough with rattling of mucus.

Phosphorus has pain in larynx, tickling cough, constriction and heat.

Sanguinaria covers cough of gastric origin; spasmodic and tickling.

Consider: *Carbo-V, Dulcamura, Lobelia, Rumex, Sambucus, Spongia, Squilla, Pulsatilla.*

As in all cases homeopathic, prescribing and determining the best-suited remedy in an emergency or epidemic situation can be difficult and challenging. Often, illness strikes without warning and preventive actions cannot be taken. In that case, the nosodes are not as effective and a complete casetaking is necessary. Symptoms based upon the totality are best, but carefully noted specific pathology and related remedies can be useful.

Match the remedy to the closest type symptoms exhibited within the illness, give the remedy in a 30c potency and wait. Too frequent a repetition of the remedy can interfere with the symptom picture and cause a relapse or aggravation.

Most of the above nosodes, when given as a prophylactic, should be taken during the first indications of the disease, and preferably when news of the disease is being spread throughout the community.

Dose as follows (with the prophylactic):

Before the disease reaches the household: 30c one time per day for three days.

When the disease is in the household: 30c, 3 times in water for a day, then once a week for 3 weeks.

If no effect with the prophylactic, consider the best-suited remedy to the illness and give a 30c in water three times per day for two days only. Repeat one time per week until improvement, and then stop.

As the remedies build-up the body's immunity to each diseased state, they provide an inner ability to combat various susceptibilities and weaknesses. Although studies have not been conclusive as to the prophylactic effect, one such study did show that when pertussin was given to 364 children as a preventive for whooping cough, none of them contracted it, despite coming into direct contact with the disease.

Another study of 82 individuals in close proximity to people infected with polio, and an additional 63 children and 19 adults in direct contact, found that after taking a prophylactic none of them contracted polio.

In yet another study, those children who maintained the required vaccination procedures, over 49 percent contracted whooping cough directly as a result of the vaccine. Measles vaccinations have shifted the age of contracting the disease to later stages in life, often with untreatable symptoms.

Additional findings from such organizations as the World Health Organization (WHO), the British Journal of Medicine and the Harvard School of Public Health have disclosed numerous health problems arising solely from vaccinations. These include AIDS, brain tumors, chronic Epstein Bar Syndrome, mutation of blood cells and an overall diminished immune system.

Homeopathy alleviates these tendencies and does so in a safe, nontoxic manner, either as a possible prophylactic or from a well-chosen remedy based upon the symptom picture.

Chapter Fourteen

Questions and Answers

Question: How does homeopathy work?

As briefly discussed earlier, several theories exist which explain the principles of homeopathy, but no one is certain how it truly works. It seems to work by stimulating the immune system or vital force, in turn allowing the organism to find its own balance and overcome diseased states or disharmonies.

Numerous double blind studies have increasingly validated the effectiveness of homeopathy, while attempting to appease the scientific community with its typical desire for theory substantiation. *How* it works has never been proven in a conclusive manner.

Every living organism is a form of energy, requiring food and liquids to survive. These foods and liquids are also energy, thus providing energy to an energetic being. Homeopathic remedies are energy which have specific signatures or pictures that reflect their essence. By determining the essence of an individual and a clearly related symptom picture, the most similar remedy to that picture will assist in releasing suppressed symptoms while establishing balance.

Much like an automobile battery that needs recharging, a remedy works to recharge the organism and allow it to reach its own level of recovery without constantly recharging. One dose will give an adequate representation of the effectiveness of that particular remedy.

When two similar energetic systems combine, the integrated result is harmony. Harmony establishes equilibrium while maintaining health and eliminating the causes of disharmony. As a helium balloon tends to rise to its highest level possible, so too will a human being when given the proper charge. If allowed to find its balance without interference, the organism will heal in its own fashion. Rather than interfere, remedies stoke the fires of healing by resonating with the vital force.

Despite scientific study and analysis over the past 200 years, a description of how homeopathy works has never been made clear. Clarity and effectiveness come from the result and the repeated "miracles" described in the texts.

So, ultimately it is not how homeopathy works, but rather whether it works. And it does, over and over again.

Question: Does homeopathy eliminate disease?

There have been cases where a medical diagnosis has established clear symptom pictures of diseased states and where they subsequently indicated that recovery was impossible. When homeopaths reviewed these cases and patients were willing to try an alternative or complimentary medicine, results were verifiable through follow-up medical tests.

To be clear, homeopathic remedies are not the eliminating cause. After taking a remedy, an organism's increased ability to heal itself establishes the necessary balance to eliminate the disease.

As previously described, pathology alone is rarely addressed in homeopathy, unlike orthodox medicine. The totality of the case is analyzed to reach a remedy conclusion best-suited for the person and not just the disease.

Casetaking that focuses solely on the disease, which some beginning homeopaths tend to do, seldom brings success. On a few occasions, a remedy that would be effective for the diseased state will also be the best remedy for the totality. The percentages are low for such a coincidence and addressing a person in this manner can be more harmful than helpful.

The harm comes from the delay in assisting someone to reestablish homeostasis while trying to eliminate the diseased state. Additional harm arises from pathological use of remedies and possible suppression of the disease. This occurs where there is an appearance of relief when in fact the disease has moved to another part of the body, without establishing a permanent cure.

A homeopath in California tells of a case where he administered the remedy Sepia because a patient had a brownish discoloration that appeared to look like a saddle and covered the bridge of her nose. However, he disregarded the fact was that Sepia did not fit her totality. He wanted to impress the patient with his ability to eliminate an unsightly discoloration and possibly get referrals in the future. Neither of these philosophies serves homeopathy nor the patient.

The woman called back in several weeks indicating that the discoloration had disappeared and that she was very pleased with homeopathy in general and the homeopath specifically. Six months later, the discoloration returned, appearing worse than before with none of the original symptoms being altered in the slightest.

In another situation, a patient came to my office for a chronic case of varicose veins, which were unsightly and somewhat painful. After taking the full case and deciding that a specific remedy would be quite useful, a dose was administered. The remedy had little relationship to varicose veins, but it did fit the person. Some six weeks later she returned to the office exclaiming that the veins had improved tremendously and she also was feeling much better.

By treating the person and not the disease, we give the body time to heal itself. Healing cannot be forced. Recovery will be unique to each individual and the time necessary for that recovery is also unique.

Question: If homeopathy can eliminate disease, can it also remove negative emotions like anger, impatience, violence and others of that nature?

Before answering the question, it is important to understand that not all diseases can be eliminated with homeopathy. If an individual has reached a state of degeneration or

debility that prevents the system from recovery, then homeopathic remedies can only help in reducing pain but will not
eliminate the disease. *Remember, the body and its ability to
stimulate recovery is the ultimate healing device, not the
remedies.*

With respect to emotional and mental symptoms, homeopathy creates balance rather than elimination. We carry
certain tendencies on the emotional sphere, whether inherited or conditioned, and these attributes are a part of our
nature. To remove them would be a form of altering who and
what we are as individuals.

For instance, a Sepia-type woman will generally be irritable, angry, overwhelmed with stress, detached from her
family, desirous to escape from loved ones, sarcastic, indifferent, depressed and often suffering from a past grief. By
giving Sepia to this type of woman, these symptoms will not
be discharged, but rather brought into systemic balance. In
this case, the symptom picture and the person will present
as softer, more caring and less overwhelmed by her emotions.

The symptoms have not been removed, just equalized. This
equilibrium can become a part of the body's ability to recover
and maintain itself on a permanent basis, but the underlying
tendency continues to exist. It has just reached its own level
of harmony.

Another factor to consider is the cause of current emotional
disharmony, perhaps a trauma or injury or even a delusion.
By touching upon this cause and relating it to a similar
remedy picture, the imbalance may very well be permanently
removed.

If a person has had a sense of insecurity their entire lifetime,
look to the underlying factors contributing to this imbalance.
Perhaps it stems from abuse as a child. The child may feel as
if they are unworthy of being loved because their parents hit
them for not listening or obeying. Or, it may come from a
delusion of abandonment, which feels real to a child, but is

in fact untrue because the parents were there, but they were not interactive enough for a sensitive toddler.

By addressing the causes of insecurity or low self-esteem, the sense that there is a lack of self-worth may very well disappear. Then the true cause may require additional work and evaluation for a different remedy. Often, the first remedy chosen will not touch the cause deeply enough to provide the balance needed to cure.

Anger is another emotion which rarely stands alone, but has a precipitating source, establishing a strong negative effect. Anger when constructively channeled has motivating properties, but far too often the anger is destructive and harmful. The feeling beneath the anger may be a need to be heard and the only manner that occurs is through frustration and yelling.

Screaming with anger may stem from the need to push someone away, in conjunction with an inability to adequately express one's needs. Or, perhaps the only means of emotional expression was experienced through family anger and the individual has been conditioned in that manner.

Beneath the anger lies insecurity, abandonment, a need to control or even deeper emotions of fear and separation. Attempt to understand the piece that exists within the emotions and the choices for a remedy become clearer.

In certain situations, remedies may eliminate the emotional turmoil, but only when there is an underlying causal aspect such as described above. The causal factor, when properly addressed with the most similar remedy will find its own balance, but remain within the organism.

Question: Can a remedy create symptoms unrelated to the individual?

On occasion, a remedy selection is so far removed from the person's totality that a proving is established and new symptoms arise which are unrelated to the existing symptom picture.

This is pure ineptitude on the part of the homeopathic prescriber. Even a beginning homeopath knows that a remedy is selected on the presenting symptoms and that there must be some relationship between symptoms and the remedy. Otherwise, a proving is inevitable.

Fortunately, provings are infrequent unless intentional. As a result, an individual will not become angry, impotent, develop cancer or create some new symptom. If a person has previously had a symptom in the past which they do not recall, it may appear to be a proving. More than likely, the body is just releasing a suppression to establish homeostasis.

People are often concerned that the remedy will cause some unforeseen disease to arise because they do not fit the entire picture of the remedy. Any similarity between the remedy picture and the person's totality will prevent that from occurring. A person can be assured that the remedies are safe.

It is a rare occasion that any remedy selection is completely identical to the presenting person's symptoms. There will be subtle differences between the two presentations and this does not prevent normal response or resonance.

Arsenicum Album has a strong picture, with its fastidiousness, fears, restlessness, selfishness, chilliness, organizational tendencies, burning sensations, avarice, anxiety, compulsiveness and dependency. If an individual has all these symptoms, then there can be no question as to the remedy selected.

Even if this person only has symptoms of restlessness, burning sensations, fears and fastidiousness, the remedy will be effective and can be used safely without worry of establishing a proving. It may not be the simillimum, but it can assist in clearing symptoms and guide the homeopath to a deeper-acting remedy.

There are situations where a person may say that new symptoms are occurring, caused by the remedy. Often, upon further questioning or questioning of the family when recollection is vague, these "new" symptoms are previously existing childhood illnesses which were suppressed. This is an aggravation in homeopathic terms and will bring about balance after being fully released. This should only take a few days if the proper potency was prescribed.

Question: How is potency determined and how often should a remedy be repeated?

Many homeopaths have struggled with potency selection and there are various factors to consider in the choice, including the centesimal or decimal potency.

Most of the health food stores sell the decimal or "x" potency, as they have been informed that it creates less aggravations and is safer. The "c" potencies are diluted 99 drops of water or alcohol to one drop of substance, whereas the "x" potencies are diluted one drop of substance to 9 drops of water or alcohol. Neither is safer or less prone to aggravation than the other.

Hahnemann primarily used the "c" potencies before embarking on the use of LM's in his later years. The LM's are made from stock 3c potencies and diluted 1 drop of the 3c to 500 drops of water or alcohol. All potencies are shaken or succussed vigorously after dilution. The "c" potencies seem to be in greatest use by homeopaths, mostly because the "x" potencies rarely go beyond a 200x and "c's" reach to 100,000c or CM.

The higher the potency number, such as the CM, the stronger the effectiveness and more powerful the remedy. The lower "c" potencies, 6c and 12c, are effective yet not as long-lasting. They often need to be repeated more frequently, even daily.

Repetition will depend on results or changes, whether for better or worse (an aggravation). If a 12c was given for a cough and the cough symptoms improved considerably, then the dose would not be repeated until those cough symptoms returned, even after 3 or 4 days. Should that same potency aggravate the cough symptoms and the person seems worse than before taking the remedy, then it will not be repeated.

The aggravation reflects that the remedy has been too stimulating for the system and any additional dosing will only cause further aggravation.

Severe aggravations indicate that the potency was too high. If the duration of the aggravation is persistent and intense, lower the remedy to the next lowest dilution to restore balance. For instance, a 30c was given with a subsequent intense aggravation. Give a 12c to eliminate the aggravation. Despite the aggravation, or healing crisis, the result verifies that the remedy selection was a good one, just too high for this particular individual. There was remedy-to-person resonance and the correct potency will bring about a cure.

Individual sensitivity is another factor in determining potency. If an individual is very sensitive to his surroundings, the environment, foods, smells or prior medications that have been taken, then be assured that they will also be sensitive to the remedies. LM or 6c to 12c potencies with infrequent repetition is best in these circumstances. Especially, when used in water dilutions.

For instance, a person who is sensitive to external sensual impressions, odors and noises but is also outgoing, open, excitable, anxious, sympathetic and generous—this would fit the remedy Phosphorus. A 200c potency given to this individual might be perfect and quite effective, yet if they have also indicated that previous medications have caused intense reactions, then a 30c potency is sufficient.

By dosing with one pellet of the 30c in four ounces of distilled water, just one time while waiting for any effect, a homeopath can ascertain the sensitivity of the individual. If no changes within three days, begin dosing every fourth day. If no effect, then one time every other day. Upon any response or change, stop the remedy until the response has found its own balance, then repeat as necessary, given the changes that resulted. Repeat as necessary suggests that old symptoms of disharmony are returning. Balance or improvement does not require repetition of the remedy.

There is no need to overstimulate. The most similar remedy to the person's totality is the key, not just the potency. Potency relates to the individual's ability to be stimulated or overstimulated. Overdosing with a high potency is unnecessary and is not what Hahnemann describes in the Organon as the "minimum dose."

In addition to individual sensitivity, vitality or energy is an important consideration in potency selection. Should chronic fatigue or low vitality be a part of the symptom picture, then overstimulation would cause an intense reaction to the remedy, creating further debility. Lower potencies, up to a 30c, are very effective in these circumstances. Again, the dose is given one time while waiting for a response from the person's system. Basically, the person's reaction reflects the effectiveness of the dose and the potency. Listen to the need of the body before repeating.

On the other hand, someone with a strong constitution who lacks great sensitivity and is of high energy may require a stronger potency, such as a 200c. There is no need to go to a 1M potency, as the 200c can be quite aggressive and effective. If a homeopath begins with a high potency, then this creates limitations as to how much higher they can go in potency selection.

Higher potencies, such as 200c, 1M, 10M and up, are not repeated frequently, maybe once every 30-40 days, but again, only as necessitated by the symptom picture. There is no hard and fast rule about repetition of any potency. The person will tell us by their symptoms when he or she requires another dose. Do not get caught up in a rigid mindset about when to repeat a remedy—use caution and be patient.

Be cautious of the person who wants to "nuke" the disharmony with a high potency in an attempt to eliminate it immediately. A homeopath tries to avoid adverse reactions from too high a dose. By educating a person about possible ill effects of a high potency, they can maintain a healing curve that best suits the vital force and not the person's ego.

Besides, rarely is a disharmony one that arose overnight. It has taken years to reach this level of illness and it will take time to recover harmony and eliminate suppressions. Health may improve considerably over a short time span, but total immediate cure is unlikely. Long-term illness that has endured over ten years may take up to 18 months to "cure" with the proper use and dosing of remedies.

Potency selection may also depend on the age of the person. Infants, toddlers and the elderly may be more sensitive or lack vitality, thus requiring lower potencies to initiate their recovery period. A homeopath increases the potency as indicated by the change in symptoms and improvement, or when the potency given no longer seems to be holding as well as it had in the past. *Be certain that a remedy picture remains before preceding with the identical remedy. Stay with the same potency as long as it continues to work. If symptoms have changed, then the remedy picture has probably changed as well.*

Higher potencies are often required for intense pain or for a severe degenerative disease. They work because they resonate with the disease, yet are artificial stimulants and higher on the energetic plane than the disease. As mentioned previously, degeneration may not be reversible. The intent in that situation is elimination of pain and suffering while allowing the personal transition to be more comfortable. Begin with a 200c and proceed as reflected by the symptoms. Pay attention to how long the remedy holds in these circumstances, as severe pain may require repetition more frequently or at a higher dose.

Higher potencies are derived from succussion which allows the liquids to retain the energetic make-up of the remedy. The lower potencies are more like a shotgun while the higher potencies are more like a laser. This means that being more precise in prescribing so as to avoid an aggravation or a proving.

Question: Is there a good time to take a remedy and what is the best way to ingest it?

Time of day for taking the remedy is not frequently addressed. Through trial and error, just before bedtime seems to be the most appropriate when it comes to constitutional prescribing. This is because the body is in a relaxed state during sleep, with no other interfering components like food, stress or relationships to hinder the effectiveness. Also, the body has about eight hours to establish a resonance with the remedy before it is bombarded by daily activities.

Obviously, this is not always the optimum situation as circumstances may prevent taking the remedy before sleep, such as an intense acute disharmony where the remedy will be taken when needed. Other situations will arise where time is of the essence and the remedy should be taken as common sense demands.

Remedies can be taken in many ways. Depending on the individual and their circumstances, water dilutions appear to be the most effective.

A water dilution is prepared by placing 1 or 2 pellets in 4 to 6 ounces of distilled water, dissolving them and then stirring well. One gulp of this mixture is taken before bedtime and then covered. It is not necessary to refrigerate, just keep it out of direct sunlight. The next evening, add more distilled water, stir well and take a second gulp. Discard the remainder. The remedy will not be repeated until needed and that depends on symptoms, potency and return of old symptoms.

Giving the remedy in water is also very effective for acute or intense pain circumstances such as teething, allergies, tooth extractions, headaches, PMS and other similar type disharmonies Prepare the remedy as above, but use a low potency and sip every ten minutes for about one hour or until the pains have diminished, whichever should occur first. Stir the remedy before each sip and add water if necessary. *Under no circumstances should the procedure go beyond one hour.*

If no effect after that time, consider another remedy in a few hours, but continue with the lower potencies.

When a remedy is having no effect on the illness, then it was not a good choice. Analyze and review the symptoms to determine another one. Some illnesses change and evolve quickly such as colds, flu or coughs. This requires frequent reevaluation of symptoms and remedy changes.

For infants, the low potency water dilutions are given by the teaspoon, but not with the above frequency. One time should give an indication of relief or the need to choose another remedy. Do not jump to a new remedy too quickly, as infants and even toddlers may require a few hours before the remedy is effective.

Other ways to give remedies include the traditional means of using the cap of the remedy vial and popping the remedy under the tongue to dissolve. Using the vial cap eliminates the need to touch the remedies and possibly contaminate them with various energies the hands have come in contact with during the day. This is called dry ingestion or dosing.

Dry dosing does not allow for as much nerve contact as water dilutions, but is the second most effective way of taking a remedy. For someone who is in a coma or unconscious, a remedy can be either placed on their skin or under the nose. By smelling the remedy, the energy will be imparted to the person in a more subtle fashion, but still be effective. Repeat the dose in water after the person wakes, should a relapse appear imminent.

Dissolving a low potency of Calendula and then placing it into a spray bottle with distilled water is effective for cuts, lacerations, incisions, rashes or other wounds and abrasions. Just spray on the area and allow to dry before placing the bandage or getting dressed. There are also creams made by homeopathic pharmaceutical companies which work well. Arnica creams, which are often just tinctures and are not potentized, should not be used on open wounds as they can be toxic in various forms other than homeopathic.

Questions and Answers

Despite the labels and directions on the homeopathic vials sold by the health food stores, only one or two pellets are necessary. Being as safe as the remedies are, a person could take the whole vial without ill effect or any type of poisoning, but just a few are all that is needed for effectiveness, even with the very smallest pellets or tablets.

Question: What's the best way to store remedies?

Remedies should be stored out of direct sunlight and in a cool, dry, odor-free area. When opening vials, avoid strong smells or perfumes, as the energy of these odors can alter the effectiveness and energy of the remedy.

Frequent opening of a remedy will also affect its potency and diminish its power. The remedy is nullified or weakened after a certain point of continued reopening, although the only total nullification of a remedy comes from intense heat.

When traveling, avoid x-ray and infrared machines and have the remedies hand checked to avoid any possible contamination. X-ray, which is another homeopathic remedy may adversely affect some remedies. Some homeopaths say that these machines do not alter the remedies, but why take the chance when traveling, as replacement remedies may not be available and hand checking consumes so little time.

Do not open more than one remedy at a time so as to avoid cross contamination. There have been stories of students who open the vial and sniff the contents to determine if the remedy is still potent. It is not recommended to smell the remedies, as this can establish a proving. Also, smelling remedies does not provide a clear indication of the effectiveness or strength of a given remedy.

Remedy vials can touch each other without concern, as long as they remain closed. One homeopath describes a person who kept a very strong essential oil in the same case as her remedies, yet had no problem with their continued ability to work.

Using common sense and realizing remedies are energy, and energy can be affected by many sources, including the environment and odors, will diminish the chance that a remedy has been altered.

Question: What is meant by antidoting a remedy?

There are several views on antidoting remedies and the responses depend on each homeopath's experience. Some say that very little will actually antidote remedies while others limit a person's intake of coffee, marijuana, medications, cocaine and many other substances.

Much depends on the sensitivity of the person and how they react to external agents. There are tales of someone walking out into bright sunlight after taking a remedy and having it antidoted. How the homeopath could know that the remedy was working in such a short time span is unknown, but questionable.

A medical doctor, practicing homeopathy in a prison, relates cases where his patients would take their homeopathic remedies with coffee, smoke marijuana, inhale strong odors from their work, yet continue to have the remedy bring about balance. Most of the remedies were lower potencies, such as 6c, and taken frequently, but were not antidoted by their choices or lifestyle.

The term antidoting means that a well-chosen remedy, which fits the totality, has been neutralized by another form of energy. The various energies that allegedly antidote remedies, include:

Coffee

Strong essential oils: peppermint, teatree and eucalyptus

Camphor

Moth balls

Nail polish and remover

Hair perms and coloring

Recreational drugs of all types

Excess alcohol

Electric blankets
Dentistry, especially drilling
Acupuncture
Medications
Intense heat
Stress
Trauma
Fright or shock
Grief

The possibility of antidoting depends greatly upon the sensitivity of the person and their response to various stimuli. This is a question asked of all individuals during casetaking. Individuals are frequently advised to eliminate or decrease the above substances from their lifestyle, at least for a few weeks. This helps to determine the effectiveness of the remedy. After several weeks, there should be some sign of the remedy's value in relation to the totality of symptoms.

If coffee should then be reintroduced into the daily pattern and symptoms return, then the remedy may have been antidoted. The best means of evaluating this possibility is through analysis of symptom changes, improvement, return of old symptoms and when symptoms returned in relation to the possible antidoting.

It would appear that remedies are extremely sensitive to many internal and external sources, but generally that is not the case. You need to realize that remedies can be antidoted, use caution with the above list and evaluate on the symptom picture before, during and after dosing. There is no need to be rigid, just aware of possibilities.

Question: How do remedies cause aggravations?

An aggravation is defined as a *healing crisis*, which means that preexisting symptoms return in reverse order of appearance. As Hahnemann has repeatedly stated, "Above all else, do no harm." So, despite the fact that a healing crisis is a normal human response, aggravations should be minimal in time.

If a remedy is given in too high of a potency, a 200c or so, then an individual who is sensitive or lacking in sufficient vital force to accept this potency, will have an aggravation. Duration depends on the severity of the previous symptoms and should last no longer than ten days. A brief aggravation releases suppressed symptoms while allowing the person to continue normal activities.

Someone has been overstimulated if an aggravation is prolonged beyond ten days. Most individuals have a difficult time enduring an aggravation that lasts beyond one day, but release is important and the dose should not be antidoted or lowered unless the symptoms are too intense.

Aggravations can be diminished by proper dosing and lower potencies, as there is no need ever to overstimulate. Analysis and evaluation of the symptom picture and the person as a whole can prevent a prolonged healing crisis.

There are several types of aggravations, ranging from the ideal to the severe. The following examples may be helpful.

A 32-year-old woman with painful PMS calls two days after taking a remedy and states that her period started and she wasn't in her normal emotional or physical pain. Aggravation in this case was subtle or slight and symptoms improved, a good sign of health and a strong vital force.

A 68-year-old man with chronic constipation has a prolonged aggravation (21 days), and no subsequent improvement after taking a remedy. Either the potency was too high and he was overwhelmed or the case is incurable. Reevaluation is necessary based upon the current picture.

If there is improvement after a long, not too intense aggravation, then be persistent with the selected remedy and potency as the remedy is on target and recovery will take time.

When the aggravation is brief, intense and rapid, this indicates a long-term permanent recovery. Should someone feel generally better, yet symptoms remain the same as before taking the remedy, it is a sign of deeper resonance and balance. Older symptoms will begin to return shortly, which is an excellent result.

After taking a remedy for migraine headaches, a woman feels much better for a week, then the migraines return. Repetition has no effect. This reflects that the remedy was a temporary palliation but did not touch the deeper cause or the constitutional state. Find another remedy or evaluate on the miasmatic level to discern an underlying predisposition.

A 22-year-old man with the flu takes a remedy and symptoms unrelated to either the present picture or any preexisting ones arise. This is a proving and the remedy selection had no relationship to either the person or the symptoms. A better suited remedy will eliminate the proving and establish balance.

Some individuals are so sensitive to all remedies that they either have a proving with each one given or have intense aggravations, despite low potencies. Consider the remedies Nitric Acid, Nux Vomica, Phosphorus, Sulphur or Arsenicum Album and determine if they fit the person so as to clear the case and bring balance.

Remember that aggravations cover both the existing symptom picture and older illnesses, such as childhood asthma or eczcema. The older symptoms often recur to a lesser degree than they were originally and pass more quickly. Inform patients about this possibility so as to avoid midnight phone calls.

Question: When two or three remedies seem to fit the totality, how do you choose the best one?

Many polycrests have similar actions, which often creates some confusion in the beginning. By studying materia medica and understanding the essence of the remedies, a homeopath can discern the key aspects of not only the individual but of the remedy as well.

To begin with, reducing the selections to two or three remedies is a good start. Read each one and see which fits the person's primary symptom picture along with their personality and history. Then review the casetaking notes to establish unusual or peculiar symptoms. These are the confirming aspects which create a clear differentiation between one remedy and another. Then look for food desires and sleep patterns to complete the evaluation. Return to the materia medica, review the finer points of the three remedies and a single one should become clearer.

This becomes easier with time, study and experience. For instance, what if the three remedies were Arsenicum Album, Nux Vomica and Phosphorus? On the surface, differences exist in each but the similarities between the person and the symptoms keep coming up in a repertory.

Each of the remedies:

Are chilly

Have respiratory problems

Are anxious

Crave alcohol

Have gastric problems

Desire company

Have various fears

Have concern for others

Have some compulsive tendencies

Are sensitive to numerous impressions

It is the differences which allow the homeopath to eliminate remedies and finalize their choice.

Nux Vomica and Arsenicum are closely related to each other with fastidiousness, restlessness, organization, compulsiveness and perfectionist tendencies. But Nux is sensitive to wind and is often troubled with constipation. They awake at 3 a.m., thinking about work, as they are frequently addicted to work and have insomnia. They overindulge in most anything they attempt and suffer the consequences. Arsenicum is sensitive to the smell of food and cold, while tending more toward loose stools or diarrhea. Their sleep is restless and they have difficulty sleeping between 11 p.m. and 1 a.m. Arsenicum's compulsiveness and organization stems from the need to be in control. Money is a very big issue, as is selfishness.

Phosphorus and Arsenicum have major fears, anxieties, concern for others and thirst. Arsenicum's fears relate to disease, robbers, poverty, cancer and they have despair about their recovery. They desire company to establish security for selfish reasons. They thirst for sips of large quantities of water.

Phosphorus fears something bad may happen or fears the dark and thunderstorms. They also have concern or fear for others. They are anxious for others because they are so caring and sensitive. They are open and sympathetic and desire company to express their joy and compassion. They are extroverted and generous. Their thirst is for ice cold water.

All three remedies have distinct food desires and sleep patterns which vary dramatically. By discovering the finer components of each remedy as well as the core essence, the final selection becomes obvious, despite the initial similarities.

If all else fails, read the remedy selections to the person and get his or her input about any unique connections between them and the specific remedies. One will stand out above the others and perhaps by reading, the homeopath will also get a clearer picture.

Question: Why are the miasms so difficult to understand? Can anything make studying them any easier?

Hahnemann's principles of miasm arose from his inability to understand why a well-chosen remedy sometimes would not work. He developed the miasm theory to account for the causes of inherited illness and predispositions to certain diseases. The ideas are derived from ancient philosophies and reflect the notion that a microorganism attacks the system and creates disharmony or disease. This diseased state, if left unattended or suppressed, establishes itself into our genetic make-up and alters our DNA. This affects not only the host individual, but succeeding generations.

The difficulty lies in the complex nature of the diseased state and the subsequent reactions of the human system. A human system in disharmony manifests symptoms uniquely to each individual and these symptoms reflect the appropriate approach for recovery. As a result, it is the individual who seeks the best-suited path for their recovery, not the homeopath.

For instance, if a specific remedy is valuable in balancing the system, then there may be no need to address deeper miasmatic tendencies. On the other hand, should several remedies only provide temporary help, then using a miasmatic approach may be helpful in clearing susceptibility to a specific disease. At that point, a return to the best-suited remedy for the totality will often provide more permanent relief.

As a general rule, miasms have unique symptom pictures, similar to remedy pictures, but in a broader sense. The three primary miasms, Psora, Sycotic and Syphlitic represent disease states of varying qualities and dimensions.

Psora is the root of all chronic disharmony, according to Hahnemann and is the result of suppression of the scabies infection or "itch." Destruction of tissue is rarely present, but skin symptoms, infection, depression, apathy, fatigue, sensitivity and chronic digestive disorders are specific manifestations of the miasm.

The Sycotic miasm represents an overgrowth of tissue as a result of suppressed gonorrhea and displays in the form of warts, tumors, cysts and moles. Fluent discharges abound in this miasm and the odor is often offensive. On the mental/emotional level, there can be cruelty, jealousy, irritability, deception and suicide.

Suppressed syphilis establishes the Syphilitic miasm with its tissue, bone and organ destruction tendencies. Mentally there is dullness, desire for solitude, poor memory, low esteem, self-destruction in a slow manner (smoking, alcohol etc.) and stubbornness.

Many of the mental and emotional aspects of the three miasms have similar components, yet it is the underlying causative piece that establishes its need or choice. Is it overgrowth of tissue or is it destruction of tissue? The answer will guide a homeopath toward the selection of the remedy or miasm.

Miasms tend to be inherited rather than established during one's lifetime. This predisposition creates weaknesses in specific areas of the body that can be triggered at various points in life through stress, sexual contact, environment, diet or trauma. The awareness of an inherited miasm is frequently limited, as few relatives discuss the sexual diseases of their ancestors. The symptoms provide the direction, not the knowledge of ancestors.

Study the miasms through their broad components and causative symptom pictures. Develop an image of each miasm in your mind and then draw a portrait of the symptoms on paper. Look for these images in your daily activities and while you take cases. When you finally have an instinctive feel for each miasm, begin to use the various remedies related to the miasm. The nosodes related to each miasm have their own symptom pictures, but it is recommended that they be used with caution in the initial stages of practice.

Despite specific presenting pictures, nosodes relate to a miasm, and suppression can occur if improperly prescribed. If a nosode should fit the totality and the cause, then a proving or suppression would be rare.

Understanding miasms will probably always be somewhat difficult but time, study and experience will establish a proper foundation. At least then it will feel more comfortable to use the miasmatic theory. This is especially true when many well-selected remedies have proven ineffective and temporary.

Question: Do remedies have any specific relation to each other? Are there some that should not be used together?

The answer to both of the questions is yes. In the back of *Kent's Repertory*, there is a table which covers the relationship of remedies, including those which follow one another well and those which create ill effects when preceded by others.

The relationship of remedies to one another is unique and often complex. A remedy such as Ignacia seems to work exceptionally well for acute grief and has a strong connection with Sepia and Natrum Muriaticum, both of which follow Ignacia when chronic disharmonies are involved. This is only true if either of those remedies suit the individual, but frequently that is actually the case.

Both Phosphorus and Causticum are for individuals who are sensitive, sympathetic, fearful, have respiratory problems and neurological disorders. Yet, it is stressed in many materia medica that these remedies should never be given in conjunction with one another. The relationship seems to cause further disharmony for reasons discovered after they were given in succession. We can learn from others miscalculations and experiences.

Remedies such as Sulphur, Calcarea Carbonica and Lycopodium, when given in that order have proven effective for all types of skin disorders, yet each has its own quality and must fit the totality before use. Otherwise, the result is limited. This is called a series of remedies, as opposed to remedies that follow well.

The individual headings under the Relationship section in *Kent's Repertory* begin with the remedy, then complementary remedies, then those that follow well, inimicals, antidoting remedies and finally, the duration of each remedy.

Complementary remedies are those that carry on or complete the previously given remedy in a successful manner. It can be a chronic complement of an acute or an acute of a chronic. Chronic remedies such as Natrum Muriaticum may have several acute complements, such as Ignacia, Apis, Bryonia and Capsicum.

The ideal is to give one remedy in one dose to determine effects and duration. In current society with the overuse of drugs, suppressions, confused miasms and inherited tendencies, complementary remedies can be useful and often required to clear symptom pictures.

The first dose of a remedy may last for months and remain the remedy of choice for years. More often, the first remedy is only palliative and a repetition may provide no further relief. At this point, the "Remedies that Follow Well" section can be useful in determining the second prescription. As with all remedy selection, the totality is the basis for choice, not just a heading.

Following well means that the first remedy has not completed the cure and a second or third remedy is needed. This section will give some direction and although they may not be the only choices available, it is a good starting point.

Inimacals are remedies which do not follow each other well, as described above with Phosphorus and Causticum. Their interaction is not harmonious and may in fact cause an antagonistic effect. Apis and Rhus Tox have this relationship, as does Nux Vomica and Zincum, Allium Cepa and Allium Sativa, Ignacia and Coffea, and Mercurius and Silica. There are numerous others and the chart should be reviewed before proceeding with the next remedy.

Remedies that antidote other remedies means just that, certain remedies will nullify the previous one given. Despite this section's intent, the designated remedies do not always have the intended effect, so this section should not always be counted on to eliminate a bad remedy choice.

Antidoting is a difficult issue and the attempt should be addressed with caution. If symptoms are new and intense, a proving has occurred. The reevaluation of the case and a better remedy will eliminate the proving, or if given in low potency it will diminish within a short period by itself.

When a remedy does not fit the symptom picture and it is chosen from the section on antidoting based on that intent alone, a new proving could occur or there could be no change at all. Find the best remedy for the person and their symptoms and the proving will be resolved.

If the remedy is not creating a proving, but was too high of a potency and caused an overreaction, then reduce the intensity by using the next lower potency. Antidoting in that event is unwarranted and may confuse the case.

Antidote with caution and clarity, do not overreact to an intense situation by attempting to nullify the remedy. Reevaluate and analyze the cause, the reaction and the new symptom picture before antidoting a remedy.

The section on duration deals with the time that a remedy will endure within the human system. In many ways, this information is unnecessary and often inaccurate. Each individual is unique and the duration of a remedy will also be unique. Some doses will last several months and others only several weeks.

Much depends on sensitivity, diet, stress, relationships, obstacles, environment and remedy reaction. What is mostly meant by duration, is the general time that each particular remedy *may* last, not necessarily how long it will last.

Remedy relationships are important and the specific connection should always be considered when choosing a remedy, especially in the event the remedies are inimical to one another.

Question: What is meant by the term "obstacle to cure?"

Hahnemann mentions this term in the Organon on more than one occasion. His reference comes from cases where a well-chosen remedy had an impact, but did not cure. He came to the realization that there might be an obstacle to the cure, and once removed, the remedy would act more deeply and permanently.

An English homeopath, Jeremy Sherr, has a wonderful analogy and story about these obstacles."Imagine that before giving a remedy, an individual is locked in a very small room and chained to a single bed, with no comforts, no windows, no toilet, no food, dirt and germs everywhere and no light. Then a remedy is given. The chains disappear, there's food, the room becomes brighter and less dirty, there's a window and a toilet and the room gets bigger."

Changes have occurred because of the remedy resonance, yet as a result of continued obstacles within the individual, they remain locked in the small room. Until these obstacles are altered or removed, complete and permanent cure is limited or even prevented.

Obstacles come in many forms and styles. Partly, it means addressing the demons within, the pieces which perpetuate negativity and disharmony.

For instance, diet can be an obstacle. By overindulging in foods, drugs or alcohol—-specifically known to result in headaches, allergies or indigestion—an individual creates his or her own disharmony. An awareness of the body and its usual reactions are good starting points. If there is a reaction to food, carefully monitor the duration and symptoms of the reaction. Reduce or eliminate the intake and reevaluate the reaction after consuming that particular food again at a later time.

Late meals, one or two hours before bedtime preclude restful sleep. The system requires time to regenerate and rejuvenate and this occurs during sleep. If late meals are continuously consumed, the person is digesting food during sleep, and is not regenerating optimally. Upon waking, there is fatigue and possible irritability. Give the body the rest it needs, eat light and early, avoid meat at dinner and limit the intake of alcohol. Occasional breaks from the normal routine are fine, but not on a daily basis.

Lack of exercise may be another obstacle to cure. Regular exercise of some sort, even daily walking, can assist a person in stimulating health and recovery. A general sense of well-being and energy will often come naturally after a regimen of regular exercise. There are situations where exercise may be too painful or impossible, but by attempting some form of exercise that is comfortable, individuals can recover their sense of hope and possibility.

Additional obstacles include poor sleep habits, coffee, processed foods, smoking, too much meat and dairy products, overwork, reliance on medications which no longer are necessary, lack of social interaction and overreaction to the stressors in one's life.

Relationships are also possible obstacles to cure if there is negativity, abuse or a lack of nurturing and love. Many individuals remain in unsatisfactory relationships out of fear, insecurity and misplaced loyalty. This is one of the more difficult obstacles, as patterns become entrenched while communication is nonexistent.

There have been cited cases where, after receiving a remedy, clear boundaries are established and communication is reopened between partners. A remedy alone cannot perform or create boundaries, but it can assist in bringing sufficient balance to begin the healing process.

The environment is another difficult obstacle, as many people are stuck in a job which prevents an adequate supply of fresh air or has them sitting at a desk without reprieve. There may be chemical pollutants around, causing symptoms to arise which were not previously present. Every human being is entitled to an environment which supports rather than endangers their health. Laws are written for this very purpose and action can be taken without recourse, even if it is necessary to do so anonymously.

Emotions are another limiting factor for recovery. Negative or unexpressed feelings create inner anxiety and turmoil, which prevent harmony. Support groups are very effective in this area and can assist in establishing lines of communication with similar suffering people. Writing about the emotional pain or cause may uncover deeper feelings and allow some understanding of current behavior. By releasing the unexpressed emotions in a constructive way, one can bring about balance on the inner planes.

Individuals require nurturing in a special way, unique to each of them. When this nurturing is lacking or prevented, self-worth suffers. The feeling of separation or depression follows and confidence diminishes even further. This can occur early in life when parents have little time for their child or later when there is loss of a loved one or mate.

We can reestablish balance within by nurturing ourselves on a daily basis. It could be as easy as writing, painting or drawing, but it is best to allow it to be on the creative level, so that the inner essence is being nurtured. By nurturing in this manner, we are basically saying that we feel we're worth spending the necessary time and effort to heal and find harmony.

When the obstacles to cure are reduced, eliminated or balanced, the human system has an opportunity to recover more fully and quickly. The body has the innate ability to heal itself and with the aid of homeopathy, the process is accelerated. And with the removal of obstacles, the process is permanent.

Question: Can remedies be categorized by personality types?

It is probably best not to categorize any individual according to type, as homeopathy seeks to discover the unique aspects rather than the common or general ones for each person.

In reality though, many homeopaths do make determinations according to "types." This includes personality, coloring, body shape, emotions and appearance. There are specific "types," but just as frequently, typecasting can be totally disregarded and the totality will point to another remedy.

For instance, Pulsatilla people are generally overweight, blond and blue-eyed. They are more often women with dependency issues who are warm-blooded, affectionate, timid, soft and have strong desires for company. Mood swings are common as is the craving for cool, open air. Pulsatilla is a hormonal remedy for PMS, headaches, vaginitis, menopause, gastric and sinus problems and respiratory disharmonies.

There are many people who fit either the Pulsatilla emotional picture or just the physical ailments, yet do not have the appearance of a "typical" Pulsatilla woman. The remedy is best given on specific need or presentation, not appearance.

Sepia is another female remedy, and although any remedy can be used for either sex, some are more predominant than others. Freckles or skin discolorations are common as is a crack in the middle of the lower lip. Natrum Muriaticum shares this symptom. The Sepia woman is tired-looking, appearing overwhelmed and exhausted, mentally dull and indifferent. They look puffy and pale and have dark circles under the eyes. Sepia is a great thyroid remedy, along with its use for constipation, chronic fatigue, grief, depression, PMS, hormonal disharmonies, low back pains, menopause and infertility.

Many remedies have their designated "types", but some are more familiar and used more frequently. Nux Vomica is one that fits this description with its characteristic "Type A" personality picture. This individual is filled with life, is always on the go and is competitive, compulsive, tense, irritable and has frequent emotional outbursts.

The Nux Vomica personality is also addictive, whether it relates to drugs, alcohol, exercise, work, food or sex. The Nux person is organized and tidy, much like Arsenicum Album, but without the extensive fears. Sensitivity is reflected in their anger and intolerance, especially over minor things. Insomnia is a large part of this remedy, primarily waking at 3:00 a.m., with an inability to return to sleep for several hours, and then waking unrefreshed. The cause is often excessive thinking about business.

Nux Vomica is an effective liver and digestive remedy, as well as a good hangover remedy.

Another liver and digestive remedy is Lycopodium, but it also fares well with kidney and skin disorders. The appearance of the Lycopodium individual—the person fits the symptom picture of a Lycopodium proving or it has been established that this type of person seems to do best with Lycopodium—is varied and far-reaching. They often have freckles on their face, a slightly red nose and flared nostrils upon talking.

The upper body and face is lean, but there is little muscular development and the lower extremities are full. One hand or foot may be cool while the other is warm and both are clammy. Thuja shares these symptoms, as do several other remedies. Emotionally they are unique in their anxiety, duality—they act differently at work with superiors than they do at home with family members—fears of failure and public speaking and temper tantrums, even as an adult.

They are also very opinionated, mostly because of their low self-esteem which results in their unwillingness to have anyone know about their inabilities or weaknesses. Clinically, the remedy covers constipation, colitis, cysts on the right side· of the body, warts, ulcers, hepatitis, herpes, eczema, impotence and headaches.

Phosphorus appears as a freckled redhead with fine hair and long eyelashes. They are slender and tall with an openness and concern that are obvious. Extremely sensitive, they are affected by all types of stimuli, including noise, odors, light, music, chemicals and the emotions of others. Generosity, sympathy, affection and desire for touching are common traits found in a Phosphorus person.

Fears, anxieties, anger and fatigue from being too sensitive also fit the symptom picture of Phosphorus. Clinical aspects include hypoglycemia, hypersensitivity, heart problems, cancer, multiple sclerosis, all types of respiratory problems, dizziness, depression, tinitus, hypertension, nosebleeds and ulcers.

To some degree or another, each remedy is related to a specific appearance or type as an aspect of its portrait, but prescribing on appearance alone rarely covers the totality. These observations can provide a valid starting point in choosing the confirming remedy. Beginning homeopaths play a typical game of typecasting people according to how they look as they pass them on the street, such as, "That's a Sulphur if I ever saw one." A fun game, but witho t merit in proper casetaking.

Question: Do the signs of the Zodiac have any relation to homeopathy and specific remedies?

Some homeopaths discuss a relationship of planets and homeopathic remedies, obviously based on their unique theories and observations. The idea is to establish a picture of the various aspects of each sign and discover corresponding remedy relationships.

One perspective discusses the twelve cell salts with the twelve planetary signs. A review of each relationship may provide some insight into any effects a remedy has on specific "signs."

Aries (March 21-April 19): **Kali Phosphoricum** is the cell salt. Symptoms include mental exhaustion with irritability, restlessness and extreme sensitivity to all external impressions. There is a high degree of sympathy for the suffering of others as well as anxiety about the future and an inability to cope with their circumstances. Physically, they have headaches, indigestion, fatigue, insomnia and diarrhea.

Related remedies: *Zincum, Gelsemium, Pulsatilla, Ignacia, Coffea, Phosphorus, Rhus Tox, Cimifuga, Hyoscyamus.*

Questions and Answers

Taurus (April 20-May 20): **Natrum Sulphuricum** is the cell salt. Symptoms include suicidal tendencies, mental confusion, fastidiousness, depression and tendencies toward overresponsibility. These are usually serious, intense individuals with a possible history of sexual disfunction or venereal disease. Emotionally they are closed, yet sensitive. Physically, there is often a history of head injury, asthma, digestive disharmonies, liver disfunction, arthritis and allergies.

Related remedies: *Sulphur, Thuja, Mercurius, Silica, Bryonia, Graphites.*

Gemini (May 21-June 20): **Kali Muriaticum** is the cell salt. The symptoms are mostly physical ones, with exception of the delusion that one will starve. Generally, there are many sinus-related activities, headaches, gastric and respiratory disharmonies, skin abscesses and arthritic type pains in the extremities.

Related remedies: *Bryonia, Mercurius, Apis, Thuja, Pulsatilla, Sulphur, Iodum, Spongia and Rhus Tox.*

Cancer (June 21-July 22): **Calcarea Fluorica** is the cell salt. Symptoms include depression, grief, concern about financial ruin, anxiety about health and indecision. On the physical plane, this remedy relates to teeth, bone, muscles and joints. Arthritic pains are well covered, as are bony growths, adhesions, sciatica, tumors, indigestion from fatigue, low back pains and croup.

Related remedies: *Calcarea Carbonicum, Phosphorus, Mercurius, Ruta, Aurum, Silica, Fluoric Acid and Magnesium Muriaticum.*

Leo (July 23-August 22): **Magnesium Phosphorica** is the cell salt. Symptoms include the typical fears of Phosphorus, forgetfulness and a tendency to talk to themselves. Their pains cause weeping and any physical or mental strain makes them feel worse. They tend to be irritable and hypersensitive, with mental dullness or an inability to think clearly. Physical symptoms include muscle cramps, neuralgia, colic, PMS, toothache, hiccoughs, whooping or spasmodic coughs, and most all pains are better with heat and pressure.

Related remedies: *Colocynthis, Gelsemium, Ignacia, Nux Moschata, Nux Vomica, Belladonna, China and Lycopodium.*

Virgo (August 23-September 22): **Kali Sulphuricum** is the cell salt. Symptoms include low self-esteem, irritability, sadness, depression, anxiety, hurriedness, shyness, and fear of falling are strong components to this remedy. Typical Kali's are conservative, moral with a somewhat rigid nature. On the physical plane, they are worse with heat, have chronic ear infections, nasal congestion, asthma, possible arthritis, allergies, skin disharmonies, including skin cancer and colicky stomach pains.

Related remedies: *Pulsatilla, Sulphur, Natrum Muriaticum, Calcarea Sulphuricum, Hepar, Silica and Sepia.*

Libra (September 23-October 22): **Natrum Phosphoricum** is the cell salt. Symptoms reflect a refined individual with similar tendencies to both Natrum Muriaticum and Phosphorus. They are extroverted, anxious, nervous, fearful, intuitive, easily annoyed and forgetful. Mental fatigue or dullness is another aspect of this Natrum. Symptoms may arise after uncontrolled loss of seminal fluids, even years afterwards. Physically, there are ailments from excess acidity or lactic acid. Asthma, hay fever, headaches, allergies, rheumatism, sexual disfunctions, heart palpitations, thyroid problems and parasites are additional symptoms.

Related remedies: *Natrum Muriaticum, Phosphorus, Calcarea Carbonicum, Nux Vomica, Staphysagria, Natrum Carbonicum and Rheum.*

Scorpio (October 23-November 21): **Calcarea Sulphuricum** is the cell salt. Symptoms include changeable moods, irritability, anxiousness, fears, loss of memory and jealousy. The symptom picture also includes a tendency to be opinionated, argumentative and controlling. Swollen glands, frequent and chronic yellowish discharges, eczema, boils, suppurating tonsillitis, chronic ear infections, nasal congestion, croup and chronic sinusitis are the common physical aspects of this cell salt.

Related remedies: *Hepar, Sulphur, Silica, Kali Muriaticum, Belladonna, Tuberculinum and Psorinum.*

Sagittarius (November 22-December 21): **Silica** is the cell salt. A person needing Silica is yielding, sensitive, obstinate, irritable, conscientious about minor details, quiet and has a poor memory. There can also be performance anxieties, indecisiveness and fear of needles or sharp objects. Excess perspiration, especially of the head and feet, is common. Also, swollen glands, chronic ear and throat infections, fatigue, bone, nail, teeth and hair deficiencies, immune insufficiency, constipation, respiratory problems, and slow development in children are typical traits. Being a major polycrest, Silica covers many disharmonies, but is centered on low self-esteem and lack of internal "grit."

Related remedies: *Calcarea Sulphuricum, Hepar, Pulsatilla, Mercurius, Thuja, Fluoric Acid and Picric Acid.*

Capricorn (December 22-January 19): **Calcarea Phosphorica** is the cell salt. Symptoms include great mental anxiety, grief, discontent with all matters, impaired memory, boredom, never feeling satisfied and a strong desire for travel are the key constituents of Calcarea Phosphorica. There is mental fatigue arising from their constant dissatisfaction with life, yet they are often friendly and emotionally open. In children, there is slow development, growing pains, headaches and teething problems. Neck, back, joint and bone pains are common, along with physical fatigue and either obesity or emaciation.

Related remedies: *Calcarea Carbonicum, Causticum, Tuberculinum, Phosphorus, Zincum, Ruta, Sanicula Aqua, Silica, Sulphur.*

Aquarius (January 20-February 18): **Natrum Muriaticum** is the cell salt. Natrum Muriaticum is another large and frequently used polycrest. Symptoms include being overly sensitive, emotionally closed because of disappointment in love, introverted, romantic and very responsible. They fear being hurt due to past grief and are offended easily. Compulsive tendencies abound, along with fears, fastidiousness, irritability, desire for solitude, sadness and a need to be perfect. Nail-biting, PMS, headaches, hay fever, cold sores, herpes, photophobia, ulcers, skin disharmonies, dryness, respiratory problems, high blood pressure and thyroid problems are the physically related symptoms.

Related remedies: *Ignacia, Sepia, Lycopodium, Sulphur, Apis, Bryonia, China, Causticum, Phosphoric Acid and Staphysagria.*

Pisces (February 19-March 20): **Ferrum Phosphoricum** is the cell salt. Symptoms include being easily annoyed with trifles, indifference, loss of hope, talkativeness, inability to express words or thoughts, mania and possible delirium are the usual mental or emotionally related symptoms. Due to its predisposition toward unclear symptoms, this remedy is frequently used at the earliest stages of colds and flus when there is not a clear symptom picture. Low grade fever, some flushing of the face, diarrhea, inflammation of the infected area, gastric and respiratory problems, sore throat and perhaps a nosebleed are the typical, yet vague, physical symptoms.

Related remedies: *Ferrum, Phosphorus, Belladonna, Aconite, Gelsemium, Rumex, Bryonia. Mercurius, Hepar and Sulphur.*

The theory behind the cell salts comes from Dr. Schussler, who felt that certain tissue components are found in everyone and vitality is dependent upon these constituents. According to Schussler, these salts are the foundation upon which we exist and when they are out of balance, the human system reflects the disharmony. He limited his work to twelve specific salts so as to provide a basis for ease of use and assimilation.

Schussler's work continues to grow and has been validated through additional provings and clinical experiences.

Chapter Fifteen

Some Final Thoughts

We live in a society that thrives on instant gratification. Fast cars, fast foods, faster computers and fast-acting medications. Each remains in constant demand. Even homeopathy has attempted to move into the 21st Century by creating remedies for the masses and their mass illnesses.

Since Hahnemann's first theories over 200 years ago, homeopathy has established itself as a means of cure unmatched in any millennium. Homeopathic principles help by discerning the uniqueness of an individual in relation to his or her symptoms. There are no quick cures or short cuts to health. The body takes months and years to reach a state of imbalance and manifest chronic symptoms, and it often takes several years to recover balance and release them.

The uniqueness of a person's system determines his or her rate of healing and no amount of persuasion will alter that time frame. Medications will give the appearance of health, but long-term side effects or suppressions are the result. Once the medications are discontinued, symptoms can return, and are frequently more intense.

Homeopathy, in its pure form, provides an energetic stimulation of the entire body. With the correct remedy in chronic cases, up to 50 percent improvement happens within the first month. The body may require many months to recover from the final 50 percent, but gradual and continued improvement is often better than recurring aliments.

On the other hand, something called modern homeopathy is being used to attempt to reach a larger group of individuals for economic reasons, much like orthodox pharmaceutical companies. This type of homeopathy is practiced by people who are unwilling to take the time and effort necessary to educate themselves about the principles of homeopathy. It is a means of using many remedies at-the-same-time, to touch a specific pathology, rather than the person as a whole.

For instance, a person with a headache can go to a drugstore, look at the titles on "homeopathic" bottles and choose the one for headaches. The bottle or vial may have from 6 to 10 combined remedies in low potency, some of which have been proven and some of which have not. The ones with true provings are frequently related to various aspects of a headache and often one of them will work. But the cause is never addressed and the headache will return, working much in the same manner as an aspirin, eliminating the effect without touching the underlying source.

Some will say that at least it *is* more natural, but should a proving arise from a combination remedy, then having it be natural may be the least of the possible problems that could arise. Is it natural to take something that has been diluted, potentized and labeled homeopathic, but does not have any proven picture of what it can cause? Not likely.

The problem does not lie with the acute prescriptions as much as with the chronic ones. Acute illnesses will find balance with or without proven homeopathic remedies, but chronic asthma or eczema need deeper and clearer remedy choices not found in over-the-counter packaging. This type of homeopathy is a disservice to all individuals interested in an alternative to conventional medicine.

Most who seek a complementary medicine do so because they have had little success with the normal avenues and are frustrated or in pain. By presenting "modern homeopathy" as a form of natural healing for both chronic and acute aliments, these companies mislead and confuse interested individuals. Their claims are unfounded and questionable.

Homeopathy has survived western medicine and individuals who have labeled it quackery. Scientific studies have shown conclusively, that homeopathy works and it has worked since Hahnemann uncovered its powerful potential.

Some Final Thoughts

With the additional ability to act as a preventative, homeopathy can be used for a longer, healthier life and not just for dealing with disease.

As the awareness of true and effective alternatives grow, homeopathy, with its record of safety and nontoxicity, will continue to create an environment of balance, health and productivity. This is an exciting time, one with unlimited possibility for both healing and creativity.

Appendices

Appendix A

Suggested Readings

A Homeopathic Love Story, Rima Handley.

Art and Science of Homeopathy, Elizabeth Wright Hubbard.

A Shot in the Dark, Harris Coulter.

Desktop Guide, Roger Morrison.

Homeopathic Emergency Guide, Tom Kruzel.

Homeopathic Medical Repertory, Robin Murphy.

Materia Medica of Homeopathic Remedies, S. Phatak.

Portraits of Homeopathic Medicines, Catherine Coulter.

Principles and Art of Cure by Homeopathy, H. A. Roberts.

The Organon of Medicine, Samuel Hahnemann.

Samuel Hahnemann, His Life and Times, Trevor Cook.

The Genius of Homeopathy, Stuart Close.

The Homeopathic Treatment of Children, Paul Herscu.

The Science of Homeopathy, George Vithoulkas.

The Spirit of Homeopathy, Rajan Sankaran.

Appendix B

Intake Form and Questionnaire

Case Record

Patient's Name _____

Address _____

City State Zip _____

Date of Birth _____

Sex _____

Married _____

Children _____

Today's Date _____

Phone _____

Occupation _____

Referred by _____

Treatment Plan _____

_____

CHIEF COMPLAINTS: _____

_____

Onset _____

Frequency _____

Duration _____

Sensations _____

Modalities _____

Concomitants _____

_____

MENTAL/EMOTIONAL

_____

_____

GENERALS

_____

_____

PHYSICALS/PARTICULARS _____

_____

ETIOLOGY: (History and Causes)
Alcoholism _____
Anemia _____
Arthritis _____
Asthma _____
Abuse _____
Cancer _____
Childrens illnesses _____
Cold sores _____
Depression _____
Diabetes _____
Veneral Disease _____
Respiratory _____
Herpes _____
Hay fever _____
Heart _____
Kidney _____
Liver _____
Miscarriage _____
Parasites _____
Fevers _____
Glands _____
Hearing _____
Taste _____
Skin problems _____
Strep _____
Tuberculosis _____
Sinus _____
Tonsils _____
Veneral warts _____
Warts/moles _____
Headaches _____
Vertigo _____
Vision _____
_____
Any other major conditions: _____

Intake Form and Questionnaire

Operations: _____

Past Homeopathic Treatments: _____

Family History of Disease: _____

Ill Effects from Vaccinations? _____
ALLERGIES: _____

Normal weight and height? _____

Exercise regularly? _____

Coffee? _____
Alcohol? _____
Drugs? _____
Tobacco? _____
Tea? _____

OBSERVATIONS: _____
Nails? _____
Tongue? _____
Appearance? _____

OTHER PHYSICALS:
APPETITE: _____
THIRST: (temperature/quantity) _____
ENERGY LEVEL: _____

FOOD: _____
Desires: _____
Sweet _____
Spicy _____
Salty _____

Homeopathic Vibrations

Eggs_____
Meat_____
Milk _____
Fruits _____
Cheese_____
Veggies _____
Fish _____
Temperature of food? Others_____
Aversions: _____
_____
Disagrees?_____
_____
Digestion? _____
_____
BOWEL: _____
_____
FLATULANCE: _____
_____
URINE: _____
_____
PERSPIRATION: _____
_____
SKIN: _____
_____
SLEEP: _____
POSITION: _____
REFRESHING: _____
DREAMS: _____
MENSES: _____
_____
SEXUAL FUNCTIONS:_____
_____
BODY TEMPERATURE: (chilly or warm) _____
_____
SEASONS: _____
SUN/MOON _____

Intake Form and Questionnaire

SEA/MOUNTAINS _____
WIND _____
OTHER: _____
MENTAL/EMOTIONAL
ANGER: _____
ANXIETY/WORRY _____

_____
Company: _____
Consolation: _____
Confidence: _____
Sympathy: _____
Excitable: (causes) _____
Fears: _____
Temperment _____
Forgetful: _____
Concentration: _____
Words/mistakes/confusion_____
Grief:_____
Impatience/irritibility:_____
Critical: _____
Jealousy/envy: _____
Distrust: _____
Guilt:_____
Self-reproach:_____
Yeilding: _____
Moods: _____
Restlessness:_____
Order/clutter _____
Sadness: _____
Sensitivity: _____
Suicide:_____
Weeping: _____
Pessimist/optimist _____
OTHER: _____
_____

Appendix C

Homeopathic Resources

Homeopathic Remedies
BHI: 1 800/621-7644
Boericke and Tafel: 1 800/876-9505
Boiron: 1 800/Blutube
Celltech: 1 800/888-4066
Dolisos of America: 1 800/Dolisos
Standard Homeoapthic: 1 800/624-9659
Washington Homeopathic: 1 800/336-1695

Books
Bodhi Tree: 1 800/825-9798
Homeopathic Educational Services: 1 800/359-9051
Natural Health Supply: 1 505/982-4071
National Center for Homeopathy: 1 703/548-7792
The Minumum Price: 1 800/663-8272

Kits and Supplies
Boiron: 1 800/BluTube
Dolisos of America: 1 800/Dolisos
Homeopathic Educational Services: 1 800/359-9051
Integrated Visions: 1 800/910-1966 (Kits)
Natural Health Supply: 1 505/982-4071
Standard Homeoapthic: 1 800/624-9659

Newsletters
Homeopathy Today
801 N. Fairfax Street, Suite 306
Alexandria, VA 22314

New England Journal of Homeopathy
356 Middle Street
Amherst, MA 01002

Resonance
2366 Eastlake Ave., Suite 325
Seattle, WA 98102

Simillimum
P.O. Box 69565
Portland, OR 97201

Schools/Education
Atlantic Academy of Classical Homeopathy
21 West 58th Street, Suite 6E
New York, NY 10019

Four Winds Seminars
187 Hillside Drive
Fairfax, CA 94930

Hahnemann Center for Homeopathic Studies
P.O. Box 4383
Boulder, CO 80306

International Foundation for Homeopathy
2366 Eastlake Ave., Suite 325
Seattle, WA 98102

National Center for Homeopathy
801 N. Fairfax Street, Suite 306
Alexandria, VA 22314

New England School of Homeopathy
356 Middle Street
Amherst, MA 01002

Homeopathic Resources

Pacific Academy of Homeopathic Medicine
1678 Shattuck Ave., #42
Berkeley, CA 94709

Organizations
Foundation for Homeopathic Education and Research
2124 Kittredge Street
Berkeley, CA 94704

International Foundation for Homeopathy
2366 Eastlake Ave., Suite 325
Seattle, WA 98102

National Center for Homeopathy
801 N. Fairfax Street, Suite 306
Alexandria, VA 22314

Glossary

Aggravation: old or present symptoms get worse in order to release.

Ameliorated: when symptoms improve or get better >.

Antidote: when a remedy is altered or nullified by some other energy form.

Aphorism: Hahnemann's term for paragraphs in the Organon.

Brain Fag: mental fatigue.

Casetaking: consultation or interview for analyzing and determining a remedy.

Dilution: the degree of remedy attentuation; potency.

Diphtheria: formation of false membrane in the throat with pain, swelling, fever, obstruction, fatigue and possible paralysis.

Essence: refers to either the person or the remedy and relates to the core.

Etiology: cause of the disease or disharmony; person's history.

Herings' Law: healing usually occurs from within toward the outside; from top to bottom and in reverse order of their appearance.

Law of Similars: any substance which causes symptoms to arise in a healthy person upon ingestion, will cure those same symptoms in someone who is ill.

Layers: this refers to various levels of trauma, injury, disease or illness.

Materia Medica: a list of remedies with specific indications for each one.

Miasm: a preexisting or acquired infectious disease, which causes subsequent breakdown of the individual; predisposition to illness.

Modality: a specific condition or situation that makes a person better >, or worse <; "She feels worse in cloudy weather."

Nosode: a homeopathic remedy potentized from diseased materials.

Palliation: when a symptom is removed or reduced on a temporary basis.

Pathology: changes in tissues or organs caused by disease.

Polychrest: remedies which have multiple uses for various symptoms.

Potency: the number of dilutions for a remedy; centisimal (c) is diluted 1-99 drops of alcohol or water; decimal (x) is diluted 1-9 drops [the first number (1), is the substance, the second character, is the liquid—6x, 30c, etc.]. LM is a newer high potency that is diluted 1-500 drops [LM 1, LM2 to LM32].

Proving: the symptoms that arise after giving a remedy to a healthy person.

Remedies: substances which have been diluted, potentized, succussed and and proven by accepted homeopathic principles.

Repertory: a compilation of symptoms, indexed according to headings; remedies are listed under each symptom described.

Rubric: another name for a symptom in a repertory.

Scarlet Fever: contageous disease; chills, high fever, rapid pulse, swollen glands and a red rash caused by a strep infection.

Simillimum: the remedy that is most similar to the totality of symptoms.

Succussion: the vigorous shaking of a remedy after it has been diluted, usually about 100 times per dilution or potency.

Symptoms: changes in the system, either observed or experienced by the individual; they are usually the signals of disharmony in an individual.

Tetanus: lockjaw, painful muscle spasms and convulsations from a toxin affecting the nervous system.

Trituration: remedies which cannot be dissolved with liquid are ground up by mortar and pestle with lactose to create a powder; this is then dissolved.

Glossary

Typhoid Fever: an infectious disease that enters the body through food or water; it affects the intestines and spleen with diarrhea, fever, red spots, fatigue and possible delirium.
Urticaria: hives or rash.
Varicella: (chicken pox) red, non-scarring eruptions; may contribute to herpes zoster in later years.
Variola: (smallpox) skin eruptions which are contagious and leave scars.
Vertigo: dizziness.
Vexation: frustration or annoyance.
Whooping Cough: (pertussis) spasmadic cough with difficult inspiration of breath and "whoop" sounds upon cessation of coughing spell.
Yellow Fever: a virus spread from mosquitos which results in chills, fever, head pain, vomiting, constipation and jaundice.

References

Allen, H. C., *Allens Key Notes*, (New Delhi: B. Jain Publishers, 1988).

Blackie, M., *Classical Homeopathy*, (Bucks, England: Beaconsfield, 1986).

Boericke, Wm., *Materia Medica with Repertory*, (Philadelphia: Boericke and Runyon, 1927).

Boericke, Wm and Dewey, Willis, *Twelve Tissue Remedies*, (New Delhi: B. Jain Publishers, 1987).

Carey, G. W. *The Zodiac and the Salts*, (Los Angeles: Carey-Perry School of Chemistry, 1932).

Clarke, J. H., *Clinical Repertory*, (New Delhi: B. Jain Publishers, 1987).

Clarke, J. H., *Dictionary of Materia Medica*, (Essex, England: Health Science Press, 1987).

Close, Stuart, *Genius of Homeopathy*, (New Delhi: B. Jain Publishers, 1993).

Dancu, David, *Natures First Aid for Children,* (Boulder: Integrated Visions, Ltd, 1992).

Dancu, David, *Travelers First Aid,* (Boulder: Integrated Visions, Ltd., 1993).

Farrington, F. A., *Comparative Materia Medica,* (New Delhi: Indian Books, 1962).

Hahnemann, Samuel, *The Organon, Sixth Edition,* (Los Angeles: J. P. Tarcher, Inc., 1982).

Hering, C., *Analytical Repertory of Symptoms of the Mind,* (New Delhi: B. Jain Publishers, 1988).

Hubbard, E. W., *Homeopathy as Art and Science,* (Bucks, England: Beaconsfield, 1990).

Kent, J. T., *Lectures on Homeopathic Materia Medica,* (New Delhi: B. Jain Publishers, 1989).

Kent, J. T., *Lectures on Homeopathic Philosophy*, (Berkeley: North Atlantic Books, 1990).

Kent, J. T., *Repertory of Homeopathic Materia Medica*, (New Delhi: B. Jain Publishers, 1987).

Kruzel, T. *Acute Homeopathic Prescriber*, (Portland: Medicina Biologica, 1988).

Mathur, K. N., *Text Book of Pathology*, (New Delhi: B. Jain Publishers, 1989).

Morrison, R., *Desktop Guide*, (Albany: Hahnemann Clinic Publishers, 1993).

Murphy, R., *Homeopathic Medical Repertory*, (Pagosa Springs: Hahnemann Academy, 1993).

Ortega, P., *Notes on the Miasms*, (New Delhi: B. Jain Publishers, 1980).

Phatak, S. R., *Concise Repertory of Homeopathic Medicine*, (New Delhi: B. Jain Publishers, 1963).

Roberts, H., *Principles and Art of Cure by Homeopathy*, (New Delhi: B. Jain Publishers, 1993).

Sankaran, R., *The Spirit of Homeopathy*, (Bombay: Homeopathic Medical Publishers, 1991).

Tyler, M., *Homeopathic Drug Pictures*, (New Delhi: B. Jain Publishers, 1981).

Tyler, M. L., *Pointers to the Common Remedies*, (New Delhi: B. Jain Publishers, 1988).

Vithoulkas, G., *Science of Homeopathy*, (New York: Grove Press, 1980).

Index

218

219

About the Author

David A. Dancu, N.D., has a Juris Doctorate in law, a Master's degree in Holistic Medicine and a Naturopathic Doctorate degree. He currently resides in Boulder, Colorado with his wife, Anne and son, Joshua. He has a private practice in both Denver and Boulder, where he also teaches at The Hahnemann Center for Homeopathic Studies.

David has written articles for *FIT Magazine, Nexus. Homeopathy Today* and *Resonance,* as well as several booklets on Travel, Children's Acute Illnesses, and Everyday First Aid. He is currently working on his second book *Alternative Therapies for Cancer.*

He has been teaching for seven years, four of which have provided Certification through a 250-hour course. David is the founder and director of the Hahnemann Center for Homeopathic Studies in Boulder. He has been on the Board of Directors for both the Pacific Academy of Homeopathic Medicine and the National Board for Homeopathic Examiners.

He can be contacted at:
The Hahnemann Center for Homeopathic Studies
P.O. Box 4383
Boulder, CO 80306
(303) 447-1966